The Clinician's
Codependency
Treatment
Workbook

(66) Self-Recovery Strategies
for Clients Who Lose Themselves in Others

Nancy L. Johnston, MS, LPC, LSATP, MAC

THE CLINICIAN'S CODEPENDENCY TREATMENT WORKBOOK
Copyright © 2024 by Nancy L. Johnston

Published by
PESI Publishing, Inc.
3839 White Ave
Eau Claire, WI 54703

Cover and interior design by Emily Dyer
Editing by Chelsea Thompson

ISBN 9781683737285 (print)
ISBN 9781683737292 (ePUB)
ISBN 9781683737308 (ePDF)

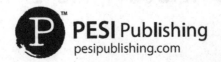

PESI Publishing
pesipublishing.com

Dedication

*For each of you who wish to live in connection with
the wisdom, strength, and serenity within you.*

Table of Contents

Introduction

Do you find working with codependency to be a clinical challenge?

Perhaps you're unclear on what it means. With no firm clinical definition, codependency often looks like a long string of descriptors that could be true of many of us at times.

Perhaps identifying codependency in clients is not within your area of focus. Even those well trained in assessing mood and relationship problems can miss the telltale dynamics of codependency and instead join the client in trying to solve the problems of others without helping them to understand and help self.

Or perhaps your challenge comes in knowing how to treat codependency once you have identified it. It's common for clinicians to refer codependent clients to self-help books on the topic or to support groups such as Al-Anon. While these recommendations can be helpful, bringing direct clinical work to this intra/interpersonal dynamic can foster substantial improvement in your client's relationship-with-self and, subsequently, with others. As this clinical work progresses, many of their presenting symptoms may be reduced or better managed by them.

In addition to feeling puzzled, ineffective, or frustrated when working with clients with codependency, you may find your efforts at treatment challenged by both popular and professional views of codependency as weak or shameful. Such views can prevent you from bringing up this issue with the client or, perhaps, seeing it in your self.

This workbook, written especially for clinicians, brings codependency out of the shadows into the clinical light of day. You will come to understand how "codependent" is not a label indelibly stamped upon a client, but rather a real intra/interpersonal dynamic that can be healed by learning to connect with and respond to self.

Some Examples

Codependency has been my specialty for decades. Both personally and professionally, it has been a theme, an area of interest, and a reason for deep growth. My personal work on codependency began in 1988 when a family member entered treatment for alcoholism. I joined a twelve-step fellowship for families of alcoholics to support that family member's recovery, not knowing that my own recovery path had begun as well. Like most people, I had no idea that my helping, fixing, and over-responsibility were part of the family system dynamics contributing to this person's addiction and to my anxiety and unhappiness.

Even as I embarked on my codependency recovery, I did not know what codependency really was. Yes, I knew the word from my training, but it was an abstract concept that described the role family members and friends can assume in an alcoholic family system. I did not understand the *experience* of being codependent, the internal goings-on that can cause emotional distress and entangled relationships.

As I worked full-time, parented, and tended to my home, only I knew how lost I felt in my primary relationships. A hint of disapproval or disagreement and I would feel like the floor just dropped out from under me. I would scramble to pull myself together by seeking affirmation and reassurance from others that, often, they could not give me. I felt anxious and fearful.

How might clients who struggle with codependency present themselves? Here are a few case examples that may be familiar to you.

> **Cynthia**, *a 50-year-old mother, has an adult daughter who repeatedly relapses from her alcohol recovery and habitually asks for help, especially in the form of money. Feeling responsible for her daughter, Cynthia worries she is not doing enough for her and fears the trouble her daughter may get into if she does not help her as she always has. As a result, Cynthia's anxiety is almost always high; she is exhausted, confused, and fearful.*

> **Jason** *is 57 years old and works a full-time job in a warehouse while also serving as the primary caregiver for his mother, who is developing memory problems. At the end of his daylight shift, he goes to his mother's home to take care of her until bedtime. Jason does not have time to be with his own children and partner or to do things he loves, like go on walks or fish. While his sister lives only 20 minutes away, she is never available to help with their mother's care. Jason feels trapped and angry, but also guilty for feeling these ways.*

> **Tyler** *is 24 years old and in her first serious relationship. After two years with her partner, Tyler is growing tired of feeling unheard by her partner and always having to do what her partner wants to do. At the same time, she feels fearful that she will be abandoned if she lets her partner know what she truly believes or wants to do. Discouraged, Tyler has lost interest in things she usually enjoys and is sleeping more than usual.*

You will get to know Cynthia, Jason, and Tyler better as we study codependency assessment and treatment throughout this workbook—they will be our case examples for applying clinical strategies. Consider them our workbook clients.

Defining Codependency

In chapter 1, we will study several working definitions of codependency in detail. Having a clear working definition is essential to good treatment. It points the way to deeper work, growth, and healing.

Historically, a codependent person has been defined as being:

- Profoundly affected by the words and actions of others (Beattie, 1987)

- Obsessed with controlling someone else (Beattie, 1987; Norwood, 1985/2008; Cermak, 1986; Co-Dependents Anonymous, 2011)

- Dependent on external sources of fulfillment (Zelvin, 2004)

- Externally focused (Dear et al., 2004)

- Lacking a sense of self (Bacon et al., 2020a)

Loss of self in others, the primary way I define codependency, captures the essence of these definitions. It is a theme, a core issue, a well-established pattern of living that permeates the client's relationship-with-self and with others. *Loss of self in others* is a real intra/interpersonal dynamic. Being dominantly other-centered, the individual loses their connection with self. They do not know how they feel or what they want and need, nor do they know how to provide these things for themselves. They may not even know that attending to self would be a good thing to do.

As the previous case examples illustrated, loss of self in others can show up in a variety of clients and can serve as a catalyst for some of the most common clinical issues—anxiety, depression, relationship problems, self-doubt, confusion, and immobility. Other clients who may lose self in others include individuals who:

- Are adult children of addicts or narcissists

- Are full-time caregivers to family members who are aging or have a chronic illness

- Have experienced relational trauma, including those who are:

  - Mentally, emotionally, physically, or sexually abused

  - In a relationship with a narcissist

  - Being gaslighted

- Feel stuck in their relationship

- Are driven to please others

- Are driven to fix others

- Need to be in control of everything

- Take care of others more than themselves

- Have difficulty saying no

Discovering this *loss of self* lens through which to conceptualize cases was therapeutic gold! As we begin doing "the work" around codependency, clients feel more connected with themselves and are able to foster a better balance in their care of self and others. They make inroads into changing their deep, long-standing patterns of self-neglect and self-abandonment. They form an attentive, reassuring relationship-with-self.

The Essential Clinical Challenge

A cornerstone of my codependency recovery has been keeping the focus on my self and not being drawn into the often complicated dynamics of the person with whom I am entangled. This focus on self is the foundational clinical challenge with the codependent client. The codependent person looks to others to know what to do, how to feel, and how to be. They make daily decisions based on the needs of others, pleasing others, or trying to control others. Their happiness and sense of self are based on things outside of self.

Codependent clients often do these things in therapy too. They may fill their counseling time telling stories about other people in their life, never getting around to self. They may seek solutions for the problems of others, having no awareness of enduring solutions for self.

There are many reasons focusing on self is difficult. You and your clients will learn to explore those reasons and develop insights and skills to help them shift from their dominant external focus to an aware and responsive internal connection. They will learn to put themselves into the formula of their lives. As they develop their relationship-with-self, they can become their own safe haven. This focusing-on-self is the fundamental shift that opens the door to self-recovery.

Self-Recovery

One day a client of mine talked about a furious argument with her partner. She was upset with him and with things she said and did. As I listened to her story of how she interacted with him in those angry moments, she seemed to be describing her own loss of self. She paused in her storytelling and exhaled. I suggested, "In your upsetness, it sounds like you lost your connection with your self and spoke and acted in ways that are not true for you at a deep, real level."

"Yes," she said, "Completely."

It was in that moment I realized, after decades of work on codependency, that this is the essence of codependency treatment: recovering our self. When we are about to physically fall down and manage to save ourselves from falling, we feel not only relieved but also capable of taking our next steps and moving on with balance and confidence. This workbook is designed to help clients learn to recover from whatever may be tripping them up or pulling them away from self and find that they can restore their connection with who they truly are.

This workbook offers a positive, growth-oriented approach to codependency treatment anchored in a model I call *self-recovery*. Self-recovery is an integrated, clinically driven treatment model that addresses the core issues of codependency: a strong external focus and a loss of self in others.

Self-recovery involves four interlocking elements: self-understanding, self-awareness, self-competence, and self-attunement.

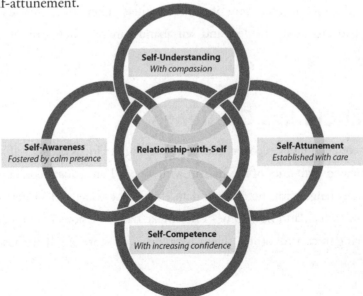

Development and integration of these four areas of growth can help clients notice and attend to self in new and restorative ways they can identify and act on.

As you use this workbook, you will be able to help your clients develop their relationship-with-self as you:

- Develop a deeper and more compassionate understanding of the core issues of codependency.

- Become more focused and confident in your clinical work with codependent clients.

- Learn practical, nonjudgmental ways to conceptualize codependency.

- Attune to the external orientation of the codependent client.

- Learn strategies to help the codependent client redirect their focus to self.

- Identify how codependent dynamics contribute to presenting symptoms such as anxiety, depression, and relationship problems.

- Help clients face the realities of self and their relationships, learn to respond rather than react, set healthy boundaries, and let go of what they cannot control.

What's in Store?
A Brief Look

This workbook offers a four-part map of clinical work that takes you through the natural progression of therapy:

I. Understanding Codependency

II. Intake, Assessment, and Early Sessions

III. Treatment: The Four Interlocking Elements of Self-Recovery

IV. Self-Recovery as a Way of Being

Within this four-part map are 66 evidence-informed strategies for codependency treatment. These strategies include everything from information to visual tools to self-reflective writing exercises. Handouts, client worksheets, psychoeducation scripts, case applications, and clinical tips accompany a number of the strategies. The handouts and client worksheets can be used by the clinician, the client, or both, during counseling time or as post-session homework. You can also use them as therapeutic conversation prompts to engage the client in the self-recovery process.

Though the workbook sections build upon each other, you can go to any strategy at any time to meet the needs or interests of your client in that moment. A detailed table of contents is provided to guide you.

A Special Note

This workbook provides a primary foundation for whatever therapy process a client may be engaged in. It offers essential information for the client who is ready to bring their focus to self and compassionately understand their tendency to neglect themselves as they focus on others.

Deeper individual therapy may be necessary for some clients. Trauma and attachment wounds are often a source of this loss of self in others. Your client may benefit from focused therapies such as internal family systems, emotionally focused therapy, somatic therapies, or eye movement desensitization and reprocessing (EMDR). Intensive individual therapy can be a part of the integrated work of the self-recovery model.

An Invitation to You

As you use this workbook with your clients, I encourage you to do the exercises too. Notice if you have tendencies to lose your self in others, perhaps through people-pleasing, avoiding conflict, or fixing someone else. I know my personal work with codependency has had a substantial impact on my professional work. Being aware of the ways I try to manage and control, make my point, or get someone else to do something invites me to quiet my self. Then I can join my client as they develop their relationship-with-self, a relationship they can trust to empower them as they live into in their self-recovery.

Part I

Understanding Codependency

Having a conceptual framework for working with codependency is essential for effective treatment. We have various definitions for codependency and lists of traits a codependent client may exhibit, *but what are we really treating?* To help answer this question, I want to share the two important influences that taught me to identify *loss of self in others* as a fundamental way to understand codependency.

My History

In 1988, when a family member entered treatment for alcoholism, I found my way to therapy and to Al-Anon, the twelve-step fellowship for family and friends of alcoholics. Tension and conflict had been a way of life for me with the alcoholic; I frequently worried about upsetting or displeasing the alcoholic and was preoccupied with fears of them leaving me. Nevertheless, I deeply wanted to make that relationship work and was willing to live with my fears and insecurities. That is, until our crisis occurred.

When I started on my recovery path, I was already a therapist with feet in both mental health and addictions. In my first job as a therapist in a juvenile corrections center with training in psychology, I quickly saw the need for learning how to also treat addictions. Little did I know that our family crisis would show me that I needed to do recovery work for my self as well. For decades I had been so focused on caring for and pleasing others that I had no idea who I really was or my part in my relationship challenges.

As it happened, the timing of my self-discovery coincided with a broader shift in clinical and cultural understanding. The term *codependency* first appeared in the late 1980s when addiction recovery and self-help were making notable inroads into our treatment approaches. Early work in alcoholism treatment identified the partner of the alcoholic as a "co-alcoholic." The co-alcoholic was described as both affected by and contributing to their partner's addiction process. As the clinical understanding of alcoholism expanded to include dependency on other substances, the term "chemical dependency" was adopted, and "co-alcoholic" became *codependent*. This term acknowledged that codependency could be present in a family member in any family system in which another member had a substance use disorder.

Early codependency treatment focused on helping the codependent understand their part in the addiction process and learn ways to support the recovery of the person with the substance addiction. This is a relevant and important focus, but fortunately, clinicians recognized that effective treatment for the codependent involved understanding who they are, what they need, and how to take good care of self in the midst of relationships with others. Several works—Melody Beattie's *Codependent No More* (1987), Pia Mellody's *Facing Codependence* (1989/2003), and others—contributed significantly to this shift toward self-focused treatment for codependents.

Another key contributor to this shift was Al-Anon. The program's suggestion that the concerned family member keep the focus on self and not the alcoholic was a watershed moment for me. Being a good daughter, partner, mother, and student was my main, externally focused way of operating. Success in these areas made me feel good; failure made me feel bad. I was not aware of my feelings and thoughts separate from the feelings and thoughts of others. Keeping the focus on my self was a revolutionary idea.

By the late 1990s, my go-to definition of codependency—loss of self in others—had taken root.

Clinical Research and Practice

Over the two decades since I learned that living with an addict invites an external focus that leads to loss of self, clinical research and practice have substantiated and extended this conceptualization of codependence. The following areas of study have been particularly illuminating on the topic:

- **Trauma:** In its early stages, codependency treatment addressed the abusive, neglectful, and chaotic living situations of the codependent. Understanding those experiences through the lens of trauma has deepened our clinical work. Trauma's impact and requisite survival skills make disconnection from self almost inevitable. By the same token, trauma healing opens the way for the desire and ability to foster self.

- **Attachment theory:** Understanding attachment styles can help us understand codependency. Some insecure attachments lead a person to repeatedly seek external validation while feeling chronically worried, fearful, or unsure, all contributing to loss of self in others. Helping clients understand their attachment styles can open the door to their creating a secure relationship-with-self.

- **Neuroscience:** The expansion of neurobiology over the past 20 years has helped us understand how activation of our sympathetic nervous system puts us out of touch with self. It has also shown us that our brain can develop new neural pathways that help us operate from a calm, confident center rather than from our survival reactions of fight, flight, or freeze triggered by trauma, chaos, and inconsistency (Hanson, 2009, 2013; Porges, 2011; van der Kolk, 2014). Helping our clients understand this biologically based process can yield profound insights that help them access their calm, centered self.

- **Mindfulness:** I have been a student of mindfulness since the mid-1990s when I first participated in Jon Kabat-Zinn's (1990/2013) eight-week Mindfulness-Based Stress Reduction and Relaxation Program (MBSR). As a result, I know firsthand the value of quieting self to connect with self. Research shows that mindful breathing and body practices can, among many benefits, decrease anxiety and stress and increase self-awareness and compassion (Hölzel et al., 2011). Through mindful presence, we can shift our awareness from external to internal, from judging to nonjudging, from resistance to acceptance—all vital ways of connecting with our true self.

The Next Era

Thanks to the advances of the last 25 years, today's clinicians are better equipped than ever to address codependency at its root: the lack of connection with self. Whether a person is attracted to people with problems or reacting due to old family roles and rules, they can be so other-centered that they are not noticing their own feelings, thoughts, and body. No blame here—as Al-Anon teaches, we did the best we could for who we were at the time. Instead of blame and regret, compassion and relief are essential for codependent people to learn about recovering self and the health that awaits them by doing so.

Thanks for joining me in learning to understand and treat codependency. Together we are moving into the next era of clinical recognition and treatment for this real intra/interpersonal way of being.

CHAPTER 1

Practical Ways to Conceptualize Codependency

In this chapter, we'll examine six strategies that are foundational to the work of treating codependency. These strategies offer clinical conceptualizations to help you understand the intra/interpersonal dynamics of codependency. In later chapters, we will expand on these concepts and incorporate them into specific strategies for self-recovery.

Strategy 1

Recognize **external focus** as a dominant characteristic of codependency.

A significant theme in this workbook is helping your client make the important shift from a dominant external focus to an attentive and responsive internal focus. Dear, Roberts, and Lange (2004) conducted a systematic thematic analysis of 11 published definitions of codependence from best-selling self-help books as well as clinicians and researchers. The analysis determined four core features of codependency: external focus, self-sacrificing, interpersonal control, and emotional suppression.

Embedded in every definition examined by the analysis, *external focus* emerged as the most important core feature of codependency. Dear and colleagues describe external focus as placing one's attention on what other people are thinking, feeling, doing, and expecting and adjusting one's self to accommodate the needs and expectations of the other person in order to receive approval and belonging. Examples of external focus include being overly focused on others, being overly sensitive to criticism, becoming emotionally dependent on others, fearing abandonment, seeking approval, having damaged boundaries with others, and basing one's happiness and identity on others. Shifting from this dominant external focus to a healthy, balanced internal focus is a primary clinical path in this workbook.

The other three core features of codependency identified by Dear and colleagues (2004) also reflect this strong tendency to focus outside of self:

- **Self-sacrificing:** Neglecting one's own needs in order to meet the needs of others

- **Interpersonal control:** Having an entrenched belief that one can fix the problems of others and control what they do

- **Emotional suppression:** Becoming overwhelmed by emotions as a result of suppressing them or having limited awareness of them

Helping our clients recognize their external focus is an important step as they begin their self-recovery work. In part II of this workbook, we will look at specific clinical ways to facilitate this process.

Strategy 2

Conceptualize codependence as **loss of self in someone else**.

Bacon and colleagues (2020a) found that individuals identifying as codependent lacked a sense of self (versus a clear, strong connection with self). Both clinical experience and research support *loss of self in someone else* as a practical way to conceptualize and work with codependency.

Handout 1: Relationship Circles is among my favorite ways to educate clients about loss of self in others. The circles demonstrate three relationship styles: enmeshed, alienated, and healthy/dynamic. Codependency recovery, illustrated by the healthy/dynamic relationship style, involves establishing an individuated circle of self that allows the client to move comfortably and confidently through interactions with others and simultaneously retain a healthy connection with self.

Relationship Circles*

Each of the following pairs of circles illustrates a relationship between two individuals, each with their own circle of self.

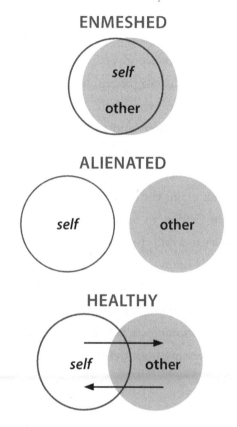

The top set of circles illustrates an *enmeshed relationship*. This relationship is relatively static, with each person holding on to the other and offering little space for their own self or the self of the other person. Notice how the overlapping selves eclipse each other.

The second set of circles illustrates an *alienated relationship*. The individuals in this relationship do not intersect—that is, they are not able to share themselves with each other. Instead, they keep their distance. They may be in the same room sharing responsibilities and spending time, but they do not come together in meaningful ways.

The third set of circles shows the individuals overlapping somewhat, yet not completely. In this *healthy relationship*, the individuals share themselves with each other while keeping a separate sense of self. This healthy relationship is not static. Rather, it is dynamic—the individuals move toward or away from each other as needed, desired, and mutually agreed upon. The circles can range from completely overlapped to completely separate depending on the honored needs of each person at any point. In other words, this healthy relationship allows for change and flow. It depends on both individuals being aware of their separateness and togetherness and wanting to foster their self and their relationship.

---

* Adapted from *Disentangle: When You've Lost Your Self in Someone Else* (2nd ed., p. 108), by N. L. Johnston, 2020, Central Recovery Press.

Strategy 3

Conceptualize codependency as **overfunctioning** in someone
else's life and **underfunctioning** in your own life.

Within the past several years, I've extended my conceptualization of codependence to *overfunctioning for others and underfunctioning for self.* This imbalance is a natural conceptual evolution from *loss of self in others.* As the codependent client becomes overinvolved in caring for, giving to, and accommodating someone else, they are simultaneously not paying attention to self. They disconnect from their feelings and needs and cannot effectively act on their own behalf.

I am not the first clinician to speak of over- and underfunctioning as important dynamics within a relationship. Family systems theory, developed by Murray Bowen (1978), maintains that individuals within a family system over- and underfunction in order to manage the anxiety within their family system. This emotional management maintains the system's status quo even if it is problematic. For example, in a case study from the Bowen Center, an overfunctioning husband completes tasks his wife had agreed to do but is not doing in order to avoid the tension and conflict that would likely come from his expecting her to take care of her agreed-upon responsibilities (Kerr, 2019).

In Bowen's work, overfunctioning and underfunctioning are treated as relationship patterns between individuals within a system. In this workbook, we will be focusing on how these dynamics play out *within one individual.* If I am overfunctioning on behalf of someone else, I am also underfunctioning on my own behalf. That is, I am generating both dynamics *within my self.* Here are some examples of what this can look like.

Overfunctioning in Someone Else's Life

- Doing something for someone that they can do themselves
- Trying to fix someone else's problem when they don't see it as a problem
- Giving something to someone when they have said they do not want it
- Volunteering to do something when your schedule is already full
- Telling another person how they feel and what they should do

Underfunctioning in Your Own Life

- Putting aside important appointments for your self to accommodate the needs of others
- Saying yes when you really want to say no
- Doing something for someone when you have already told them you won't do it
- Offering money or time you can't afford to give
- Developing anxiety, depression, or regrettable anger as a result of your preoccupations with someone else

Recognizing this imbalance offers a clear platform from which the client can make adjustments that support an improved balance in care of self and others.

Strategy 4

Conceptualize codependency as being dominantly **other-centered**.

In 1991, I wrote a graduate school paper entitled "Diagnosing Codependence" that proposed we conceptualize codependency as a pervasive pattern of *other-centeredness*. Working with literature current at that time, I explained that the other-centered person may sacrifice their own needs for those of others, think obsessively about and try unreasonably to control the behavior of others, and allow their identity and self-esteem to be governed by the opinions and feelings of others.

We are all familiar with the descriptor *self-centered*. At the other end of the continuum, other-centeredness is the active agent when a person is overfunctioning for others and underfunctioning for self. Let's take a brief look at this self-centered/other-centered continuum:

Self-Centered/Other-Centered Continuum

Self-Centered ⟵ ⟶ **Other-Centered**	
Is dominantly focused on their own needs, feelings, and perspective	Is dominantly focused on the feelings, needs, and perspectives of others
Places unreasonable demands and expectations on others	Places unreasonable demands and expectations on self
Feels entitled	Feels unworthy

As we work toward self-recovery, we are not trying to become self-centered, as some clients fear as they begin this work. Rather, the clinical goal is to be able to operate in a range around the balance point of this continuum.

Strategy 5

Consider codependency in terms of **specific behaviors** associated with codependency rather than the label *codependent*.

The word *codependent* can mean different things to different people. Some people even object to the word, believing that it blames and shames individuals for extending self to others. For this reason, I often work with codependency in terms of behaviors rather than the term *codependent*. By looking at specific behaviors associated with codependency, the client is able to understand what they are doing that may be causing problems for self and others and what behaviors they can adjust for growth.

In their textbook *Substance Abuse: Information for School Counselors, Social Workers, Therapists, and Counselors*, Fisher and Harrison (2018) also advocate speaking in terms of behaviors associated with codependency rather labeling the client. They explain that such behaviors are not good or bad in and of themselves. Sometimes those behaviors are purposeful, appropriate, and satisfying for all; other times, those behaviors can cause problems. Helping a client identify the specific behaviors involved in their over- and underfunctioning creates a clearer, nonjudgmental, actionable treatment focus.

So what are some specific behaviors associated with codependency? The following list is a compilation of behaviors cited in various definitions of codependence (Bacon et al., 2020a/2020b); Beattie, 1987; Black, 1981/2020; Cermak, 1986; Fagan-Pryor & Haber, 1992; Mellody, 1989/2003; Norwood, 1985/2008; Wegscheider-Cruse, 1989; Woititz, 1990) and itemized in inventories used to measure codependency (Dear & Roberts, 2005; Fischer et al., 1991). The listed behaviors have also been identified by individuals engaged in therapy, workshops, and retreats focusing on codependency.

Behaviors Associated with Codependency

- Giving
- Fixing
- Caregiving
- Helping
- Serving
- Problem-solving
- Working hard
- People-pleasing
- Conflict-avoiding
- Thinking for others
- Speaking for others
- Taking over
- Controlling
- Doing for the other person what they need to do for themselves

It's worth noting that not all individuals who lose themselves in others act in the same ways. Some may be very controlling and demanding; others may be caregiving problem-solvers. Some present a number of these behaviors. Moreover, I am sure there are other behaviors that could be added to this list. Helping the client identify the specific behaviors that promote their loss of self in someone else can be clarifying and point the way to change.

Strategy 6

Place behaviors associated with codependency on a **continuum**.

As mentioned previously, most behaviors associated with codependency are not unhealthy in and of themselves; we can just carry them too far. Fisher and Harrison (2018) explain that such behaviors can range from lesser to greater degrees of frequency and intensity. Seeing these behavioral gradations on their own continuum helps us to assess and treat each client.

This also helps address a common criticism of the term *codependency*: that it shames people for doing natural, loving things such as helping, caregiving, and problem-solving. The self-recovery model believes that offering these caring behaviors can be important, appropriate, and enriching. The clinical problems come when those same behaviors extend themselves into overdoing for others and undercaring for self.

Handout 2: Codependency Behaviors Continuum illustrates how an individual's behaviors associated with codependency can range from acceptable, normal, or appropriate to compulsive, destructive, or addictive. At the "okay" end of the continuum, the behaviors are normal, acceptable, and, in fact, desirable for healthy and appropriate social engagement.

The "too far" end is where behaviors associated with codependency become compulsive and addictive. The individual moves in this direction when they give beyond what they have to give, to the point that they become exhausted, irritable, angry, and increasingly obsessed with the other person. They do what they said they would not do for the other person. They think of the other person all of the time and strategize for them. They lose sleep, friendships, family, and opportunities for self because they are consumed with this other person. At this extreme, the individual has lost control of self.

If we are honest, we often know when we are moving in this direction. We can feel it in our emotions, our actions, and in the reactions of others. Rather than waiting until we have gone too far, there are things we can learn to regulate our self along this continuum. As you move through this workbook, you will learn strategies to help clients become aware of where they are on this continuum and adjust self in the direction of health.

Codependency Behaviors Continuum*

Any particular codependent behavior can be examined along this continuum:

Okay ←	→ Too Far
Keeps connection with self	Loses connection with self
Is able to be flexible and open	Is rigid, obsessed
Causes no impairment in functioning	Causes impairment in functioning
Holds a secure relationship-with-self	Holds an insecure relationship-with-self

---

* Adapted from *Disentangle: When You've Lost Your Self in Someone Else* (2nd ed., p. 54), by N. L. Johnston, 2020, Central Recovery Press.

Cynthia and Hints of Codependency

When Cynthia arrived for her intake interview, she was upset over an argument she'd just had with her adult daughter, Jenna. Jenna was in the third week of her most recent treatment for alcoholism, having relapsed three times over the past two years. Cynthia could hardly focus on the intake questions. She kept talking about her daughter's view—that Cynthia is wasting her time and money by coming to counseling. Jenna told her mother that she needs some extra money during this early phase of her recovery. When asked about this, Cynthia agreed with Jenna and wondered if in fact she should wait to begin counseling until Jenna was in better shape.

I listened fully to Cynthia and asked if she would be willing to tell me a bit more about what brought her to our first session, inviting her to remember things now obscured by her recent tangle with her daughter. Cynthia did her best to answer my questions, but she had great difficulty keeping her focus on her self. Instead, she easily shifted into telling me about her daughter's addiction and relapses, her repeated requests for Cynthia's help and all the things Cynthia did for her, such as paying her bills and cleaning her room.

Cynthia said all of this made her very anxious. She worried she was not doing enough for her daughter, that Jenna was right in blaming her for not offering enough support. She was also afraid of the trouble Jenna might get in if she did not stay close to her and provide the direction and resources Jenna demanded. Cynthia said she had become so confused and exhausted that she made this initial appointment with me because she could not think of anything else to do.

I reinforced Cynthia's belief that counseling may be a good thing for her. I explained that if she chose to continue our work, we would work at a pace that was comfortable for her in getting to know her situation and what she wanted for herself. Cynthia half-chuckled and said, "I have no idea what I want."

Cynthia rescheduled, saying she wanted to try at least one more session. She said it felt odd and good to have a calm conversation with someone who was interested in her and didn't yell at her.

Insights and Intentions

Consider the strategies introduced in this chapter:

1. Recognize **external focus** as a dominant characteristic of codependency.

2. Conceptualize codependence as **loss of self in someone else**.

3. Conceptualize codependency as **overfunctioning** in someone else's life and **underfunctioning** in your own life.

4. Conceptualize codependency as being dominantly **other-centered**.

5. Consider codependency in terms of **specific behaviors** associated with codependency rather than the label *codependent*.

6. Place behaviors associated with codependency on a **continuum**.

What have you learned in this chapter about codependency?

_____

_____

_____

Which strategies in this chapter seem particularly useful in your work with codependent clients?

_____

_____

_____

Have you had any realizations about your self?

_____

_____

_____

Are there strategies from this chapter that you might intentionally bring to your practice or into your own life?

_____

_____

_____

CHAPTER 2

Broadening Your Lens to Include the Codependency Paradigm

I've had clients refer to their codependent relational dynamics as the way they are "programmed" or as a "running code" that plays into most of their thoughts, feelings, and behaviors. By bringing that "code" into awareness, clients can make significant changes for self that reduce and manage their presenting symptoms, which often include anxiety, depression, and relationship problems.

In this chapter, you are invited to broaden your clinical lens by expanding the ways you think and feel about codependency.

Strategy 7

Understand that codependent behaviors are learned, adaptive responses to family and life experiences.

We may see client behaviors such as giving, fixing, or controlling as human behaviors that are simply part of a client's story, rather than as clinical issues. Failing to connect their relevance to the issues the client is seeking help for, we might make suggestions to modify those behaviors in some way without realizing the depth of those patterns within the individual.

Codependency is rooted in any number of experiences or events that may have happened to the person over their lifetime; its related behaviors are learned, adaptive responses to family and life experiences. (We will be exploring these influences on self-development in detail in chapter 6.) **Handout 3: Circles of Influence on Self-Development** is a concentric circles model you can use with your clients to help them understand what causes them to lose self in others.

The circle in the center represents the individual's innate nature and tendencies. Those qualities and tendencies are directly affected by the individual's family systems, illustrated by the second layer encircling the individual. Some of the family systems dynamics we will explore with the client include individuation versus fusion, family rules and roles, attachment styles, trauma—any and all factors that can affect an individual's sense of self and the extent to which they value, attend to, and respond to self. Along with the individual's family of origin, their family system may include deep-seated influences from their intergenerational family systems.

The third encircling layer in this diagram represents the broader worlds in which the individual was raised. Social, cultural, political, and religious influences can help societies to function and stabilize, but they can also restrict an individual's access to self. Through self-recovery, we are not trying to change any individual's beliefs or faithfulness to their family, church, or social structure if those things are valuable to them. We are helping them understand the sources for their deep patterns of self-abandonment, compassionately accept those patterns as important ways of survival, and decide whether and how they would like to change those ingrained patterns by establishing their relationship-with-self.

Circles of Influence on Self-Development

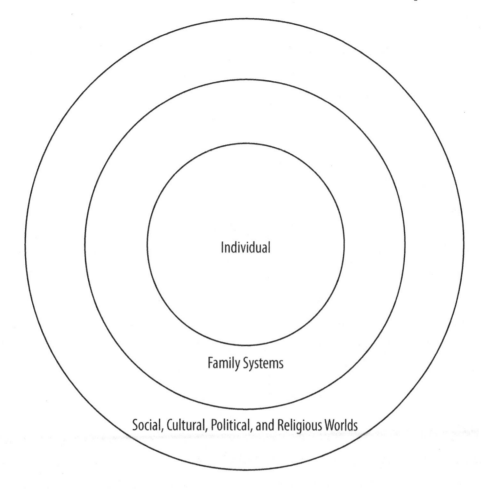

Individual

Family Systems

Social, Cultural, Political, and Religious Worlds

Individual influences: Your individual influences are at the core of this diagram. This includes who you are genetically and biologically, your innate nature and tendencies apart from the influence of the outer two circles.

Family system influences: These influences include both family of origin experiences and intergenerational family influences. Here you are looking at what happened to you when you were growing up and how those experiences remain with you. This brings up a number of factors for consideration, including family roles and rules, attachment styles, and trauma.

Social, cultural, political, and religious worlds: These can be powerful influences on the individual and on the family system. This circle invites you to examine your cultural experiences and the teachings and values of the worlds in which you were raised.

As you well know, these concentric circles bleed into each other. The details in one layer likely affect its neighboring layer. Your innate nature was no doubt affected by the way you were treated in your family. The parenting you received was no doubt influenced by the worlds in which your family was living. Still, studying each of these influences on your development of self will help you make more sense to you.

Strategy 8

Work with codependency **nonjudgmentally**.

We do not usually judge people for their anxiety, depression, or other emotional and behavioral symptoms they present to us. We simply assess and design a treatment plan with them. However, sometimes codependency can invoke judgment, blame, and shame both from the clinician and the client. Some interpret it as a weakness or as too broadly defined to mean anything important to mental health. Some view it as inappropriate helping that the individual should simply stop doing. Some even blame the codependent person for the problems of others, leaving them burdened by guilt and shame, with no space or compassion for self.

In working with the codependent client, we don't want to suggest that the behavior changes they make toward self-health are obvious or easy. We don't want to harm our client's sense of self by being surprised by or disapproving of what they think and do. Rather, we want to listen to them and help them make their own determinations about their thoughts, emotions, and behaviors. Our modeling nonjudgmental discernment will help them develop that ability for self.

When we meet the codependent client where they are without judgment, we set a healthy stage for assessment, understanding, and work together. When we bring our curiosity, kindness, and openness to them and their work, we are giving them the space to do the same for self.

Strategy 9

Identify codependent dynamics in a **variety of clients**.

Codependency is not limited to those living with other people's addiction. Losing self in someone else can present in any setting where one person is overfunctioning for others and underfunctioning for self—such as caring for children, helping aging parents, or sustaining an intimate partnership. Disconnection from self can be a primary way of operating, or it can develop as an adaptive strategy to cope with stress or trauma. Either way, our clients' presenting problems can be significantly impacted by their not being able to safely listen to and respond to self. Recognizing this underlying other-centered dynamic can be particularly helpful in their healing.

To help you recognize general patterns and behaviors that point to codependency as possibly being part of a client's total clinical presentation, let's look at Jason's early experience in treatment.

Jason and Undercurrents of Codependency

Jason entered counseling because of his chronic unhappiness and, until recently, unexpressed anger. A reliable, well-liked employee at the warehouse, Jason had an argument with a coworker when they asked if he could cover a shift for them. "Nobody gives a crap about me," he fumed. "It's always 'Jason will do it!' Well, Jason has had it! No more Mr. Nice Guy!" He stormed off and left work. The next day, his supervisor asked to meet with him to discuss what happened. The meeting ended with the supervisor asking Jason to participate in counseling sessions offered by his workplace's employment assistance program (EAP) to help him with his emotions and behaviors.

Jason attended the three free EAP sessions and wanted to continue counseling, so he was referred to me. In our early work, Jason unloaded some of the burdens he was carrying: a full-time job, a full-time family, and care of his elderly mother, who struggled with memory problems. He also spoke about his tangled relationship with his sister, who lived nearby but was never available to help with their mother's care. Jason and I approached some of these issues through problem-solving and resource development, but I invited him to take a deeper look at some of the undercurrents that might be in play and contributing to his stuckness and exhaustion.

With curiosity and active listening, Jason and I began to look at his family history. Jason was the one coming through for his mother no matter what, while his sister appeared not to help at all. Perhaps understanding old family patterns might create the possibility of change within Jason. And perhaps these patterns reflected codependency in Jason. Was he losing himself in any or all of these stressors in his life? Was he doing too much for others and not enough for self? Could Jason benefit from focused self-recovery work?

Insights and Intentions

Consider the strategies introduced in this chapter:

7. Understand that codependent behaviors are **learned, adaptive responses** to family and life experiences.

8. Work with codependency **nonjudgmentally**.

9. Identify codependent dynamics in a **variety of clients**.

What have you learned in this chapter about broadening your lens to include the codependency paradigm?

_____

_____

_____

Which strategies in this chapter seem particularly useful in your work with codependent clients?

_____

_____

_____

Have you had any realizations about your self?

_____

_____

_____

Are there strategies from this chapter that you might intentionally bring to your practice or into your own life?

_____

_____

_____

Part II

Intake, Assessment, and Early Sessions

Good work! You have completed part I of this workbook, which brought you onboard with strategies to conceptualize codependency, broaden your assessment lens, and bring nonjudgment to your work with codependent clients. Now let's get to the nuts and bolts of assessing for codependency and study visual tools to educate your client about codependency if your assessment finds they will be helped by this information.

Here are a couple of important things as we begin part II.

First, use your standard intake procedures and forms with your clients as you assess for codependency. The material in this workbook is designed to enhance what you already do. I will be sharing my intake process with you, but you are invited to decide how you would like to incorporate assessment for codependent dynamics into your own intake work.

Second, remember that we are not trying to officially diagnose codependency. Such a diagnosis does not exist in the American Psychiatric Association's (APA; 2013) *Diagnostic and Statistical Manual of Mental Disorders, Fifth Edition* (*DSM-5*). We are assessing for when, where, and how codependent behaviors and dynamics are contributing to the symptoms the client is experiencing. Paying attention to these core intra/interpersonal ways of being sheds light on beliefs and patterns within the client they may want to change in order to have lasting relief from their anxiety, depression, guilt, stress, or distress.

Let's start now by welcoming your client into your safe and calm therapy room and joining them with your full presence and readiness to know who they are.

CHAPTER 3

Assessing for Codependency in the Intake Process

The strategies offered in this chapter are best understood within the context of how I gather intake information with a client. I use an intake interview process with three broad sections: the client's presenting problems, family and social history, and mental status.

Within each of these three intake sections are important topics the client and I explore. I am interested in the specific presenting problems that prompted them to come to therapy and how those problems are affecting their mood, behaviors, and health. In the family and social history section, I gather background on the client's family of origin, including their family history of medical, psychological, or addiction problems. We also begin to gently explore experiences of abuse, neglect, or trauma. The mental status section includes the standard list of questions ranging from sleep and appetite to mood, suicidal thinking, and substance use.

My intake process is both structured and organic. I have these three areas of information and assessment to gather, *and* I want to do this work following the client's lead as much as possible. I explain my intake process to my client by saying:

Just as a portrait painter may start with sketches of a person and develop their image by adding texture, color, and detail, such is our intake process. Initially, we gather basic information ranging from who is in your family to how well you sleep. We are sketching you. We will touch on topics and later circle back to them to add important details that make your self-portrait accurate and complete. We will share this getting-to-know-you process, and I trust that we will both know a great deal about you and your needs by the end of it. We will have created a rich and meaningful picture of you that will guide us in our work together.

Strategy 10

Invite the client to **center in self** from the beginning of your intake evaluation: "What brings you here today?"

When the obligatory paperwork is completed, including the release of information and emergency procedures, I smile, set those papers aside, and invite the client to begin telling me what led them to seek therapy at this time—in other words, their presenting problem (or problems).

"So what brings you here today?"

This question helps the client connect to the reasons they set up—and kept—this appointment. It cuts straight to *their* focus:

"I am not sleeping at all."

"My partner just left."

"I just left my partner."

"My doctor told me I need counseling."

Such statements immediately give us information to explore. I am interested in the who, what, when, and where details of their presenting story, as well as the ways it is affecting them in mood, energy, and behaviors. They likely see me as an authority figure with the answers to their problems; I invite them to connect not just with me but also with self, right from the start. I want to hear from them. I want them to listen to self and to learn to value and trust self. What they say matters. What they want is important.

To support this client self-engagement, I take handwritten notes during my time with the client, often writing down their actual words as opposed to paraphrasing or interpreting what they have said. Paying attention to the client's words helps me understand and validate them. Often, I reflect their words back to them to let them know I hear them or to check my accuracy in understanding them. Our clients can get to know self more clearly and honestly as they hear their own words and clarify what those words really mean to them.

I also invite client self-engagement from the beginning by explaining how we will set their therapy goals. I say:

I am sure you have some ideas of what you want to get out of counseling, but I prefer that we set your treatment goals together later in the intake process. I first want to travel the paths with you that brought us into the room together. By the time we have talked about the information in the three sections of my intake interview, your goals will naturally be clear to both of us. We will have arrived at them together.

Strategy 11

Take the **client's lead** as much as possible.

The client and I will cover everything on the intake form, but apart from the mental status section, it will not be in the order written. Instead, the other sections are completed as our conversations flow. I do this because our clients' seemingly casual statements, questions, reflections, and requests for reassurance tell us important information about self. I want to hear, acknowledge, and explore these self-revelations with the client as they happen.

By taking our time with the intake interview, the client and I are establishing our therapeutic relationship and starting treatment even as we do this information gathering. When we have completed their intake portrait, our work is underway. The client feels heard and known. We are on the same page. Our work together feels manageable and hopeful.

Strategies 10 and 11 are particularly important as we assess for codependency. Much of what I suggest in these strategies is simply good therapy practice. We listen to the client, let them know we hear them, and foster their voice as they recover self. Most of us have been trained in the importance of these practices; still, if we are not mindful, we can lose track of them as we listen to a client's story and instead pursue various topics about their lives that catch our attention. Because of our clinical experience, we may believe we understand what is going on with our client and jump in too early with suggestions and plans. In our efforts to be helpful, we are not joining the client where they are. We are missing our connection with them by changing tracks or getting ahead of them.

These cautions are particularly important when working with a client who may have codependency. Such a client arrives with a strong external focus, ready to listen to an authority figure, eager to be told what to do, and geared toward people-pleasing. Often such individuals are in relationships in which their voice is not welcomed or is outright negated. All of this has contributed to their external orientation in protection of self. Experience has taught them that to think for self and express those thoughts may be dangerous; it may prompt conflict, harm, or abandonment. As therapists, we want to be sensitive to these dynamics and gently offer new space and opportunities for the client's voice.

Codependency can also express itself through controlling behaviors. Clinicians may experience clients who are impatient with the paperwork process, want to completely manage how and when they share intake information, or tell the therapist what will or won't work for them before the intake process has even begun. These, too, are adaptive responses that protect the self from danger. In meeting such a client, our attentive listening and readiness to join them where they are is very important to the intake process. If we seem to be telling them how they are or what they might do to help self, their issues with control may be activated. We may then find our self having a difficult conversation with them long before we have established a relationship with them.

Whether we are meeting an individual with compliant or controlling codependent tendencies, I suggest we convey our intention transparently: "I want to know who you are, what brings you here, and what you would like from me."

Jason's Intake Interview (An Excerpt)

THERAPIST: *Welcome, Jason. I am glad you are here today. We have finished all of the papers I need you to read and sign. I'm ready and glad to start getting to know you through this interview. I will be asking you questions about things that are important for me to know, and I know you have things you want to make sure to tell me. We will work on this interview together, each taking the lead at times.*

JASON: *What do you mean I will be taking the lead at times?*

THERAPIST: *I mean that what you have to say to me is very important. You may mention a topic or person that I would like to know more about, so we will go in that direction in our conversation for a* *while. I like to think of this intake interview as sketching a picture of you. At first, we may just outline certain areas of your life; later, we will go back and color them in more. I will be taking handwritten notes as we talk to make sure I am hearing you accurately and you feel heard and understood.*

JASON: *Okay.*

THERAPIST: *I like to start with this question: What brings you here today, Jason?*

JASON: *My mother. I just don't know what to do. She needs help. I give her help. But it's just not working.*

[**Note to Clinician:** Jason just gave us a great deal of information. In his five sentences, he has opened up our conversation in a number of important ways. Building from Jason's very words, the clinician could choose to go in several directions, such as more information about his mother and her needs, his "not knowing what to do," his feelings about things "not working"—all of which are ultimately important.]

THERAPIST: *Tell me about your mother.*

JASON: *She's sick, alone, and someone needs to be with her. Her memory is not good. She leaves stove burners on, forgets to eat, and wanders in the neighborhood sometimes. She can't drive, can't keep her own appointments, and just really needs to be taken care of like a little kid.*

[**Note to Clinician:** I would likely ask Jason a few questions about family history at this point—not extensively, as I don't want to move too far away from the authenticity of what he is sharing with me. I want to stay close to his very words. I want just enough information to start understanding *his* story.]

THERAPIST: *Jason, could you tell me a bit about your family? Let's just sketch them in here for a few moments. How old is your mother and how is it that she lives alone?*

JASON: *My mother is 82. My father died 22 years ago in an automobile accident. My mother was a homemaker her entire life. My father took care of most everything outside of the house. He made and controlled the money. My mother always seemed a bit afraid of him. Amazingly, she was fine living on her own after his death until her memory problems showed up a couple of years ago.*

[**Note to Clinician:** I could ask Jason more about his father and his death. This is important, but not now. I want to stick with what Jason has reported to me about "things not working" for him as he helps his mother and about "not knowing" what to do at this point.]

THERAPIST: *Okay, so that's when she started to need help? You said she needs help.*

JASON: *Yeah, lots of help, like I said. It's scary for me when she doesn't have someone in her home to watch out for her. We have someone there during the day. I come over after work, cook dinner, and see that she gets to bed. So far, she is alone through the night and nothing has happened to her.*

THERAPIST: *I notice you said, "We have someone there in the day." Who does "we" include?*

JASON: *Oh, I shouldn't have said "we." That's not true at all! "We" should be me and my sister, but it's not. I can't get her to help me in any way with Mom. She won't stay with her. She has no money to help pay for her care. She doesn't even want to help me plan Mom's care. She says, "You are so good at that. I trust you to do whatever you think is best." Sometimes she doesn't even return my texts about Mom for days!*

[**Note to Clinician:** Once again, he has offered an introduction to more important family history. I note this to myself; we will get back to his sister. For now, though, I choose to reflect Jason's feelings and explore more about what is "not working" for him.]

THERAPIST: *I hear you, Jason. That sounds frustrating and disappointing. Am I hearing you right?*

JASON: *Yup! And you can add "mad" to that list. I am just mad. This is how it has always been—"Jason will do it! You can count on Jason to take care of things!" That used to be okay with me, but now it just pisses me off! And then I feel bad that I am pissed off. I'm a mess, aren't I?*

THERAPIST: *Well, I am quite glad you are here. These are the reasons you are here with me. I appreciate your honesty. Your awareness and honesty are great starts to our work.*

Strategy 12

Assess for **codependent presentations and patterns**.

The assessment tools that follow are informal and conversational but can be quite "diagnostic." Use them within the context of your usual intake process as indicated. Remember, we are not trying to formally diagnose codependence. Rather, we are assessing for underlying intra/interpersonal codependent dynamics that may be contributing to the client's presenting problems. Identifying these long-standing patterns can promote foundational changes within the client.

There are a few formal codependency assessment tools available, including the Holyoake codependency index (Dear & Roberts, 2005), the composite codependency scale (Marks et al., 2012), and the Spann-Fischer codependency scale (Fischer et al., 1991). These tools offer a measurable score for your client's degree of codependency. The items on these scales can be used as prompts for helpful clinical discussions.

However, in my intake process, I assess for codependency using the tools in **handouts 4–8**, for the simple reason that I prefer a narrative, interactive assessment format. I enjoy exploring with the client their codependent behaviors, the extent of their codependency, and the ways it is active in their lives. As we do these assessments together, the client comes to understand what codependency is and its relevance to our work.

Strategy 13

Watch for **behaviors associated with codependency**.

In strategy 5, we talked about working with behaviors associated with codependency as opposed to the noun *codependent*. Behaviors are more specific and concrete than a broad, abstract label. Looking at behaviors can help your client see what they are doing that may be contributing to the problems they have come to therapy for.

Handout 4: Assessing for Behaviors Associated with Codependency can be used as a checklist as you gather intake information, or you can formally complete it together with the client. The handout provides space for examples of the behaviors the client engages in and their frequency. At the bottom, there are also spaces for you and your client to identify other behaviors associated with codependency specific to them. Be mindful not to judge the identified behaviors and ratings. Even seemingly supportive comments such as "Wow, you really can overdo it!" or "That just seems like too much to me" can influence your client's sense of self and obstruct their internal focus. This is simply data to help you and your client understand them more fully.

Assessing for Behaviors Associated with Codependency

Note examples of your client's behaviors and their frequency as they tell their stories. Frequency can be noted to the left of the behavior and rated on a 10-point scale, with a score of 1 meaning they mentioned the behavior once, 5 indicating they mentioned the behavior often, and 10 showing they constantly spoke about that behavior.

Frequency　　　　**Behavior**

_____ **Giving**
Example: _____

_____ **Fixing**
Example: _____

_____ **Caregiving**
Example: _____

_____ **Helping**
Example: _____

_____ **Serving**
Example: _____

_____ **Problem-solving**
Example: _____

_____ **Hard-working**
Example: _____

_____ **People-pleasing**
Example: _____

_____ **Conflict-avoiding**
Example: _____

_____ **Thinking for others**
Example: _____

_____ **Speaking for others**
Example: _____

_____ **Taking over**
Example: _____

_____ **Controlling**
Example: _____

_____ **Doing for the other person what they need to do for themselves**
Example: _____

Other behaviors associated with codependency shared by your client:

Frequency   **Behavior**

_____ _____

            Example: _____

_____ _____

            Example: _____

_____ _____

            Example: _____

_____ _____

            Example: _____

Strategy 14

Watch for a **dominant external versus internal focus**.

Helping our clients increase their internal focus opens the doors to self-recovery. First we must determine the extent to which they are externally focused. External focus can present as dominant other-centeredness or imbalances in care of self versus other.

Often, we listen to our clients tell stories about the people in their lives. They need to. They must. But do they have difficulty shifting from their stories about others to how those stories may be affecting them? When they are asked "How is this affecting you?" or "Could you tell me why this is an important topic for you today?" they may falter at this redirection. That is understandable, especially if this is a big shift for them.

Our asking is not just for the content of what they might say but also to note their access to self in that moment. It would not be unusual for a person with codependency to respond with an external focus, such as "They need help!" or "This person is crazy!" Again, it is clinically useful for us to know who and what our client is living with, but we also want to assess their ability to step away from their storytelling about others and connect with their own thoughts, feelings, desires, and needs. **Handout 5: Assessing for a Dominant External Focus** consists of a list of observations that can help you tune in to your client's ways of thinking and experiencing the world in order to assess the extent of their other-centeredness.

Assessing for a Dominant External Focus

As you conduct your intake interview, here are some themes you may note—these can help you determine whether your client has a predominant external focus.

Does your client:

☐ Talk a lot about other people and their problems?

☐ Seem preoccupied with figuring out other people?

☐ Want to fix other people?

☐ Often ask, "What should I do?"

☐ Often ask, "What do you think?"

☐ Show excessive worry about other people who can take care of themselves?

☐ Not know what to say when you redirect them back to self with questions such as "What would you like?" or "How is that for you?"

☐ Seem to be in foreign territory when invited to keep the focus on self? Seem blank or lost?

☐ Quickly shift the conversational focus back to someone else?

☐ Seem unaware they are shifting the focus away from self and back to someone else?

☐ Show resistance to considering self?

☐ Show ambivalence about considering self?

☐ Express guilt for considering self?

Handout 6: Self/Other Balance Scale is another visual tool to assess your client's tendency to attend to self/internal versus other/external. The scale illustration reminds us that the clinical goal is balance between self and others, not one extreme or the other. And as is true with a physical act of balancing, this balance between self and others involves active maintenance that self-recovery will help your client learn how to do.

The first part of the handout is a general assessment of how much your client focuses on the thoughts, feelings, behaviors, and needs of others and how much they are able to focus on those same things for self. As you assess, pay attention to whether they naturally return their focus to self. If they need to be prompted to bring the focus to self, pay attention to how they respond to your invitations to do so.

The items listed at the end of the handout consider specific codependent behaviors that indicate the client's intentions for coming to therapy. Are they there to help others? To help self? Both? Once again, our evaluation should include no judgment of what we find is true for them. We just want a sense of their focus and expectations as we begin.

Self/Other Balance Scale

SELF/ INTERNAL FOCUS		OTHER/ EXTERNAL FOCUS

In General:

_____ Needs

_____ Wants

_____ Feelings

_____ Thoughts

_____ Actions

_____ Spirit

In General:

_____ Needs

_____ Wants

_____ Feelings

_____ Thoughts

_____ Actions

_____ Spirit

More Specifically:

_____ Concerned about self

_____ Wants to figure out self

_____ Interested in fixing self

_____ Problem-solves for self

More Specifically:

_____ Preoccupied with others

_____ Wants to figure out others

_____ Interested in fixing others

_____ Problem-solves for others

Strategy 15

Watch for **overfunctioning for others/underfunctioning for self**.

The self/other balance scale leads us directly to this strategy. **Handout 7: Assessing for Overfunctioning for Others/Underfunctioning for Self** is a two-part checklist that identifies specific ways your client's self/other balance may be off.

The first part asks questions that reflect overfunctioning for others. Simply asking these questions can shed light on behaviors that the client has never considered as problematic. Most of the items involve codependency-associated behaviors that fall on the "too far" side of the behavioral continuum (see strategy 6, including **Handout 2: Codependency Behaviors Continuum** [p. 12]).

The second part of this checklist contains questions that reflect underfunctioning for self, which I describe as the opposite side of the coin from overfunctioning for others. We want to understand the ways our clients extend themselves for others *and* the specific ways they abandon self in the process. Your client may be aware of their self-neglect yet remain focused on what they feel they must do for others. Looking at how they put self aside or even shut self down is powerful and essential to their healing.

Assessing for Overfunctioning for Others/Underfunctioning for Self

This handout will help shed light on your tendencies to overfunction for others or underfunction for self. If you identify with 3 or more of the items in either or both categories, you likely tend to overfunction for others/underfunction for self. Noticing when these patterns arise and how they manifest will help you identify what to tackle first. For example, improving your ability to say no when you really mean yes (underfunctioning for self) can make it easier to resist doing something for someone when they are capable of doing it themselves.

Overfunctioning for Others

Do you:

❐ Do something for someone when they are capable of doing it themselves, such as making phone calls, scheduling appointments, cooking meals, or paying bills for them?

❐ Try to fix someone else's problem when they don't see it as a problem?

❐ Give something to someone when they have said they do not want it?

❐ Volunteer to do something when your schedule is already full?

❐ Problem-solve for others when they have not asked for that help?

❐ Take action on behalf of another person without their agreement, such as calling about a job for them or speaking with their boss about a work schedule adjustment they need?

❐ Finish the other person's sentences?

❐ Tell the other person how they feel and what they should do?

❐ Finish something the other person has not yet completed, such as yard work, laundry, or cleaning up their room?

❐ Control the household without considering the input of others living there?

Underfunctioning for Self

Do you:

- ☐ Put aside important appointments for your self, such as medical appointments or time with friends, in order to accommodate the needs of others?

- ☐ Say yes when you really want to say no?

- ☐ Do something for someone when you have already told them you won't do it?

- ☐ Offer money or time when you really can't afford to give that much?

- ☐ Offer money or time when you feel resentful about it?

- ☐ Fail to consider your self in decisions and planning, and instead simply go along with what others want?

- ☐ Become anxious, depressed, or angry when you are preoccupied with someone else?

- ☐ Lie for another person?

- ☐ Hide the extent to which you are trying to help someone else?

- ☐ Make sure the needs of others have been met before considering how you are feeling and what you might need?

Strategy 16

Recognize **codependent patterns** in various relationships and over time.

As you gather intake information with your client, watch for codependent patterns in various relationships and over time. Is your client's overextension of self to others a single, necessary event or do they tend to focus on others on a frequent basis? All of us have times and life situations when, for necessity or pleasure, we overcommit and lose self in the process. In such cases, we are usually able to retrieve our self and restore our self/other balance. In this assessment process, you are trying to determine whether your client functions in this self-restorative way or has a pervasive pattern of other-centeredness and indeed has lost self in someone else.

Handout 8: Assessing for Codependent Patterns explores your client's codependent behaviors in two dimensions: in different relationships and over time. Often, the client's codependent behaviors are not restricted to a single relationship but show up in many of their interactions with others. For example, if the client has a tendency to overfunction with their partner, it is likely they will do the same at work or with friends.

Looking at codependency over our client's lifetime is also helpful. Because their focus outside of self may be an adaptive style, we want to assess for its presence as early as childhood and adolescence. We ask about our client's relationships with their family members when they were growing up—Who needed care and who gave the care? How was conflict managed? How were household tasks accomplished? We also learn about their family history of addiction, abuse, neglect, or trauma. This information may naturally reveal the seeds of our client's tendencies to take on the needs of others to the exclusion of their own.

In chapter 6, we will use **Handout 3: Circles of Influence on Self-Development** (p. 17) to extend and deepen our client's self-understanding. For now, though, we are sketching the portrait of the client, knowing we will color in more areas every time we are together. As you conduct your intake interview, simply note when, where, and how your client's codependent tendencies have presented themselves over their lifetime and the benefits and costs of their extension of self for others.

Assessing for Codependent Patterns
In Various Relationships

With family members (e.g., parents, partners, children, extended family members):

_____

_____

_____

_____

_____

With friends (past and current):

_____

_____

_____

_____

_____

_____

With coworkers (past and current):

_____

_____

_____

_____

_____

_____

With strangers (e.g., volunteering, charitable work, activism):

_____

_____

_____

_____

_____

Over Time

As a child:

_____

_____

_____

As an adolescent:

_____

_____

_____

As a young adult:

_____

_____

_____

As an adult:

_____

_____

_____

Currently:

_____

_____

_____

Strategy 17

Identify how the client's **presenting problems may be related to codependency**.

In my experience, people rarely enter counseling because they are concerned about their codependency. They come for anxiety, depression, and relationship problems with partners, children, coworkers, extended family, or friends. They seek help for issues with food, substances, trauma, self-sabotage, confusion, or stuckness. Most of the time, they are unaware of how a dominant external focus may play a role in their presenting problems.

By the same token, I don't go looking for codependency in my clients. Rather, codependency tends to present itself through the client discounting self, showing difficulty focusing on self, or expressing guilt or resistance when asked to bring focus to self. Once I notice these patterns, I pay more attention to the possibility of codependency as an underlying dynamic.

The intra/interpersonal dynamics of codependency can be seen as personality characteristics that influence our clients' choices, behaviors, moods, and relationships. Personality characteristics cannot necessarily be identified at the beginning of therapy. Clients initially present with the issues that prompted them to seek help, but it is not until we spend several sessions with a client that we start to pick up on personality characteristics, which may include dependency, rigidity, grandiosity, or emotional instability. Keeping our lens open to notice and assess for personality characteristics makes for solid, comprehensive treatment.

The following excerpt from Jason's intake interview illustrates this identification of codependent characteristics underlying his problems with sleep:

THERAPIST: *So how is your sleep?*

JASON: *My sleep is not so good, but I know why. I don't consistently follow the good routines that help me sleep.*

THERAPIST: *Good routines. What are those for you?*

JASON: *I sleep better at night when I walk at lunchtime or at least go outside.*

THERAPIST: *What's keeping you from doing those things?*

JASON: *Not saying no to my friends at lunchtime. They are happy staying inside and eating together. I would rather eat outside and go on a walk, but I don't want to tell them that.*

THERAPIST: *What keeps you from telling them what you would like to do? Or just doing what you would like to do?*

JASON: *Oh, I don't want them to think I don't care about them or don't want to be part of their group. I want to be a good team player. I don't want to upset them and their routines.*

In just a few conversational exchanges with Jason, we went from assessing his sleep to hearing these other-centered reasons for not attending to his good sleep routines. As we entered this conversation, I had no idea where we would go. But we landed at this important topic of balancing self and others. Seeing codependency in such a concrete way creates the potential for deeper clinical work, deeper than simply reviewing sleep hygiene with Jason. Our clients often know what they need to do for change, but being able to take those identified actions involves treating the underlying "code" running within them.

The following callout shows my reflections on Jason's presenting problems and codependent behaviors, based on his complete intake interview.

Jason's Intake Interview and Codependency

Even at the beginning of his intake interview, Jason was already giving me a great deal of information about imbalances in his life. The imbalances were, in fact, the reason he came for counseling, though he did not see it that way as we started. He was extending himself for his mother's care while his sister "would not help in any way with Mom."

The phrase "Jason will do it!" offered a hint that this might be a long-standing pattern of Jason being the responsible one. The mixed emotions evident in the way Jason repeated this phrase suggested that this pattern was not necessarily okay with him.

In light of this information, I screened for codependency as we gathered his intake information. I noted his external focus as he told his stories—he was upset with others and not aware of what he might be able to say and do on his own behalf. I also noted that his way of helping others bore the signs of compulsivity—he was not able to stop himself or imagine other ways of taking care of the demands in his life.

Unsurprisingly, Jason "scored" high in overfunctioning for others/underfunctioning for self. His over-doing for others was obvious, but the checklist highlighted ways he was neglecting self, and he found the self/other balance scale to be a helpful picture. Jason became tearful as he settled into this honest self-awareness. Feeling comfortable in my presence and grateful to be heard, he finally had a bit of space for self. He also expressed doubt about being able to make changes within self to experience more balance. After all, in his words, "this is the way [he had] been for years."

Jason's family and social history explained his long-standing patterns of loss of self in others—patterns created to adapt and protect self in his family of origin. Some important details:

- *Jason was the older of two siblings. His sister, Anna, was three years younger.*

- *Jason's father died in a drunk-driving accident. His father was the drunk driver. He ran into another car on a bridge coming home late one night. No one else died in the accident.*

- *Jason's father's drinking had been a problem Jason's entire life. His father was mean and controlling when he was drinking. He never got physical, but he could be unkind and scary.*

- *Jason's mother, whom he is now caring for, was a good homemaker who tried to stay out of her husband's way. She accepted what her husband said and did, and she told the children to do the same.*

- *Jason wanted to keep the peace in the family. He tried to make light conversation, get good grades at school, and be helpful to his mother, who always had something for him to do. His constant helping at home kept him from doing the things he needed and wanted to do for self, such as completing homework and spending time with friends.*

- *Jason's sister mainly stayed in her room or away from home. Neither parent said much about this. They basically left her alone. They knew they could count on Jason to help, resolve conflicts, and be nice.*

- *Jason volunteered for community groups such as the food pantry and the homeless shelter. He said he enjoyed caregiving opportunities and would do more if he had the time.*

Synthesis: *Jason was a pro at getting things done. He was also reaching his limit on taking responsibility for others. He was not consciously aware of his imbalance in care of self and others, but fortunately, he was aware of his exhaustion, anger, and entrapment. This self-awareness was a great start, as was his willingness to remain in counseling. Through our intake he got a glimpse of his dominant other-centeredness, which manifested in his tendency to be of service to others to the minimization of self. With this realization, he started to understand how his strong external focus was an important part of the unhappiness and anger that had brought him to counseling.*

Strategy 18

Set goals *with* the client: "What would you like to get from our work together?"

Goal setting is important for bringing therapy into focus, providing markers of progress, and offering touchstones that the client can use to reorient themselves when therapy seems wandering or stuck. Wandering and stuck can be part of the process, but I find it important to know where our process is headed. And I want the client to be the primary director of what they want for self.

I set goals with the client the session after we complete their intake interview. With many of their important stories, symptoms, and history sketched in, their therapy goals are clear and waiting to be named. The client and I have done this portraiture together and are usually in agreement as we list their goals.

I introduce goal setting by saying:

Next week we will be setting your goals for therapy. You have gotten to know me some and have been willing to share what brings you here to counseling. This week, think about your goals, and we'll write them down when we are together again.

The following session I ask my client, "What would you like to get from our work together?" Because of the work we have already done to help them center in self, they are often able to express goals that connect with their personal needs, desires, and voice:

- I would like to worry less.

- I would like to be in a better mood.

- I would like to feel more energy.

- I would like to sleep better.

- I would like to know how to deal with _____.

- I would like to do less _____.

- I would like to do more _____.

- I would like to stand up for myself.

- I would like to leave my relationship.

- I would like to say no.

- I would like to express my feelings better.

- I would like to control my temper.

As clinicians, we have all written goals and objectives, and I know that each of the examples listed can be written in more objective, specific, measurable terms as needed. Most important, though, is having a clear, concrete picture of what the client is seeking for self. You can certainly add to, clarify, enrich, or help to further define any goal suggested by the client. Goal setting is a mutual process that honors the input of both the therapist and the client. That said, I suggest that the client be in agreement with any edits or additions to their goals. Their goals need to be true for them in order for self-recovery to take hold.

Jason's Goals

Jason and I mutually agreed on three counseling goals with objectives that encompass work with the four elements of self-recovery: self-understanding, self-awareness, self-competence, and self-attunement.

Goal 1: *Understand and respond to self in considerate, caring ways*

- *Study his family patterns and relationships*

- *Notice and work with parts of him that perpetuate his patterns of overfunctioning for others/ underfunctioning for self*

- *Learn to listen to the four areas of self: body, mind, emotions, and spirit*

- *Learn to make adjustments on the self/other continuum toward health*

- *Develop a supportive relationship-with-self*

Goal 2: *Improve mood*

- *Learn to calm self so as to be responsive, not reactive*

- *Develop a better balance in care of self and others*

- *Learn to ask for help*

- *Learn who can and will help*

- *Learn to set healthy boundaries*

- *Develop reliable resources for his mother's care*

- *Understand and manage his guilt*

- *Get more sleep*

- *Walk*

Goal 3: *Enjoy his life*

- *Fish*

- *Have more time with his children and partner*

- *Feel less stressed at work and when caring for his mother*

- *Explore new things he has been curious about and might enjoy doing*

Insights and Intentions

Consider the strategies introduced in this chapter:

10. Invite the client to **center in self** from the beginning of your intake evaluation: "What brings you here today?"

11. Take the **client's lead** as much as possible.

12. Assess for **codependent presentations and patterns**.

13. Watch for **behaviors associated with codependency**.

14. Watch for a **dominant external versus internal focus**.

15. Watch for **overfunctioning for others/underfunctioning for self**.

16. Recognize **codependent patterns** in various relationships and over time.

17. Identify how the client's **presenting problems** may be **related to codependency**.

18. **Set goals *with* the client:** "What would you like to get from our work together?"

What have you learned in this chapter about assessing for codependency in the intake process?

_____

_____

Which strategies in this chapter seem particularly useful in your work with codependent clients?

_____

_____

Have you had any realizations about your self?

_____

_____

Are there strategies from this chapter that you might intentionally bring to your practice or into your own life?

_____

_____

CHAPTER 4

Helpful Early Psychoeducation to Set the Stage for Change

The themes of this chapter are *educate, illustrate, invite*—all things we offer the client from the beginning of therapy.

Even as we are doing our intake interview, psychoeducation is present. We ask about worry and explain what we mean by our question. We ask about trauma and help the client understand what this may include and why we are asking. It can be the same with codependency. If in our clinical assessment we notice the presence of a dominant external focus and codependent behaviors that may be moving into the "too far" range, we let the client know what we are seeing. We introduce codependency as loss of self in others and engage them further by using the assessment tools in chapter 3.

We can also offer focused, interactive psychoeducation about codependency. We acknowledge the symptoms that brought the client to therapy and then help them see the ways codependency is related to those symptoms. We explain that codependency is not bad in and of itself; it's just that going too far in our codependent behaviors can mean losing a healthy, wise connection with self. We show how this disconnection can lead to symptoms such as those they are seeking help for. Educating your client about the interrelatedness of their symptoms and codependency sets the stage for deep, lasting change.

Strategy 19

Educate about external versus internal focus.

The following script can help you teach clients about external focus and why it is a hallmark of codependency.

Psychoeducation Script
External Versus Internal Focusing

Here's a bit of information to help you understand codependency.

A group of researchers (Dear et al., 2004) wanted to identify the core features of codependency. They studied 11 definitions of codependency used by popular writers and clinicians. They found four core defining features: external focus, self-sacrifice, interpersonal control, and emotional suppression.

In particular, external focus was found to be in all 11 definitions. What do we mean by external focus? External focus means placing one's attention on what other people are thinking, feeling, doing, and expecting, and adjusting one's self to accommodate the needs and expectations of the other person in order to receive approval and belonging.

That's a lot of words, so let's break this down a bit more.

The first part of external focus is about paying attention to the feelings, needs, thoughts, and expectations of other people in order to know what is going on with them. Now, there's nothing wrong with doing that up to a point. However, external focus is about going too far, not only in the amount of attention you are paying to the other person but also what you do with the information you are gathering by focusing on them.

The second part of external focus suggests that you are focusing on the other person so you can adjust who you are, what you think, and what you believe in order to accommodate or please the other person. In other words, you slip away from your self to be the person you believe they would like you to be.

The third part of external focusing suggests that you change your self in order to receive the approval of the other person and feel like you belong. Remember, these are normal human desires, so there is nothing wrong with wanting and seeking them. The going-too-far part is when we disconnect from our self and our internal experiences in order to please others and avoid having them be upset with us or perhaps even leave us.

The other three core defining features of codependency—self-sacrificing, interpersonal control, and emotional suppression—also involve focusing outside of your self.

Codependency treatment is about finding and maintaining a better balance in your focus on self and others. This involves developing your internal focus so your external focus is not in full control. Self-recovery is a treatment path that can help you with this balance. We will talk more about self-recovery as we work together. For now, know that the goals of codependency recovery address the four core features of codependency described previously:

- Bring your focus to your self

- Take care of your self

- Manage and control your own life

- Express your self

Recognizing your tendencies toward external focus is an important beginning of your healing process.

After presenting and discussing this script with your client, you can give them the following **Client Worksheet 1: External Versus Internal Focus** for use in session or as homework.

External Versus Internal Focus

Study

External focus is a core feature of codependency. What do you understand about external focus? Make a few notes about what you are learning about it.

_____

_____

_____

The following list includes examples of external focus. Remember, most items on this list are normal human behaviors and needs that we can carry too far. Please draw a check mark next to the examples that are true for you.

- ☐ Overly focused on others
- ☐ Overly concerned about others
- ☐ Overly sensitive to criticism
- ☐ Overly identified with the feelings and experiences of others
- ☐ Emotionally dependent on others for approval, feeling okay, security, identity
- ☐ Preoccupied with fear of abandonment by important people in your life
- ☐ Great difficulty maintaining boundaries with others

Self-Reflection

Do you feel that you may have an external focus?

_____

_____

_____

What are some other examples of ways you focus more on others than on your self?

_____

_____

_____

What are some reasons you focus outside your self? Do you have specific fears, concerns, or protective reasons for your external focus?

_____

_____

_____

As you attend to others, how might you be losing your sense of self? Can you feel this happening in the moment?

_____

_____

_____

Notes to Self

_____

_____

_____

_____

Once we have introduced the concept of external versus internal focus, it is helpful to educate our clients about what internal focus looks like. A central way I work with self is illustrated in **Handout 9: Four Areas of Self**. In this diagram, each circle represents an area of self that merits listening and response: body, mind, emotions, and spirit. The circles intersect in the diagram to illustrate how these areas of self are interrelated. Health improves as these areas are noticed and responded to.

The illustration in the handout can be used dynamically. For example, a client's circles may be different sizes, depending on the extent to which they pay attention to each area of self. Some circles may not intersect but instead be disconnected; for example, the client may be aware of their emotions but not attending to their body, overthinking, and not accessing their spirit.

Share **Handout 9: Four Areas of Self** with your client and use the following script to educate them about this illustration. Then **Client Worksheet 2: Four Areas of Self** can be used in session or for homework.

Psychoeducation Script
Four Areas of Self

We each have four areas of self that are important to pay attention to as we increase our internal focus. We have other areas of self as well, but noticing what is going on in these four major areas is especially helpful for knowing better how to respond to self, both in the moment and as we move through our day. Let's look at each of these areas.

Body: Our body has many important messages for us. Often, if we listen, we can notice that our body is sending us messages even before they register as thoughts or emotions. Listening to our body means paying attention to our physical sensations: What am I aware of in my stomach, neck, back, and face? The body gives us information through its stillness or movement: Do I feel stuck or restless? Am I moving toward or away? Listening to the body also includes the care we give it: Do I have physical complaints I am ignoring? Am I consistent with getting medical and dental checkups? Could I use a haircut or a massage?

Mind: Much of our thinking is focused on self, others, and our situations. Our thinking can be logical and rational; it can also be off-base. It can be helpful and necessary, enabling us to figure out a variety of things. But we can sometimes get lost in our thoughts and tune out the other three areas of self.

Emotions: Being able to recognize and name emotions is an important part of self-recovery. We will be working on this skill later in more detail. Here, we are simply recognizing the importance of attending to our emotions and the information they can offer us. What am I feeling? What is the assortment of feelings I am having? How do I feel about that person? That opportunity? That change of plans? Without bringing our feelings into awareness, we may well act out our emotions or eat them and later regurgitate them in some way that surprises us.

Spirit: Our spirit is just as important as the other areas of self. However, we often make decisions and take action without listening to this valuable part. Our spirit may manifest as our gut feelings or intuitions, which are strong and clear yet defy easy explanation. Our spirit may manifest as quiet mindfulness that rests our mind and emotions, allowing pieces of our life to come together in ways we could never have imagined. Our spirit may be thought of as our contact with something beyond our self, to which we can release our tight hold on a person or situation and entrust with how things unfold.

It is amazing how much information about our self is right here with us, all the time. We just have to tune in to each of these areas of self and patiently listen to what our body, mind, emotions, and spirit are telling us. Our self-recovery work will then help us know how to respond to what we hear.

Four Areas of Self*

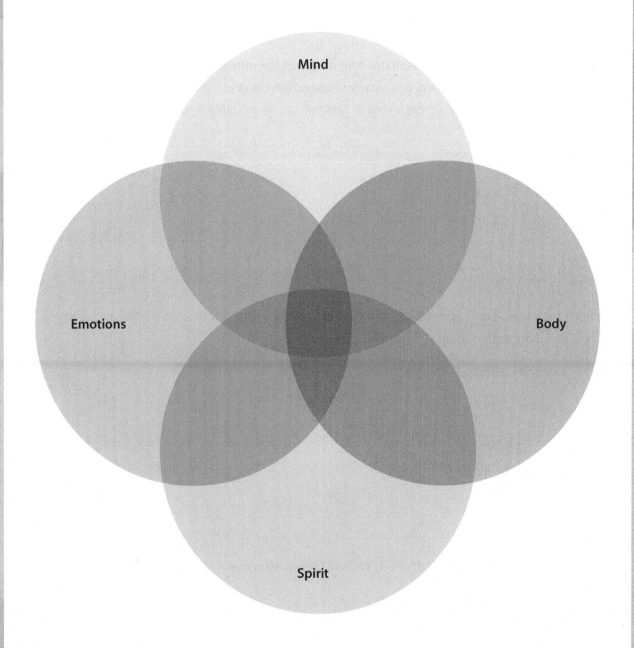

Mind

Emotions

Body

Spirit

---

* Adapted from *Disentangle: When You've Lost Your Self in Someone Else* (2nd ed., p. 160), by N. L. Johnston, 2020, Central Recovery Press.

Four Areas of Self

Study

Take a look at **Handout 9: Four Areas of Self**. Absorb the picture and the information you have been given about these four areas of self.

Do you have one or two areas that are more dominant than the others? Which ones are they? What are your less dominant areas? Are there any areas you pay no attention to? Remember, there is no right answer here. Your answers are simply meant to help you become more self-aware.

_____

_____

_____

_____

Self-Reflection

We don't have to wait until something major happens to begin listening to self. So in this moment, without self-judgment or editing (if possible), consider these questions:

What is your body telling you?

_____

_____

What is your mind telling you?

_____

_____

What emotions are you aware of? (It's likely you will find an assortment of feelings.)

_____

_____

Can you tap into your spirit? Are you aware of its presence? Can you sense any messages from it?

_____

_____

Take a moment to review what you are hearing from your four areas of self. You don't have to do anything with what you hear unless you really want to. Your practice here is to simply listen to self in an intentional way.

Notes to Self

_____

_____

_____

_____

Strategy 20

Illustrate codependent dynamics using visual tools.

Illustrating as we educate means using visual tools to teach our clients about codependent dynamics and help them further assess their codependency. Working with tools such as the relationship circles, the self/other balance scale, and the continuum, you and your client can understand the extent of their codependent behaviors and how those behaviors may be contributing to their presenting problems.

These tools can also help you set and assess the client's therapy goals. As they develop their internal connections and ultimately their relationship-with-self, how would their relationship circles interact? What would their self/other balance scale look like? Where would they be on their continuum of behaviors associated with codependency?

Strategy 21

Use the **relationship circles** diagram.

Handout 1: Relationship Circles (p. 7) is a valuable tool for early psychoeducation. I use these relationship circles with clients in several ways. I draw the diagram on a flip chart, whiteboard, or piece of paper, or I make circles out of colored plastic file dividers. These circles can be various colors and sizes. In workshops, I usually provide materials for participants to make their own circles. In my office, I keep a set of plastic circles nearby for the client and me to hold and move around to illustrate the relationship dynamics as we talk. This hands-on tool helps the client understand self in relationship with others, set their treatment goals in describable ways, and imagine connecting with and strengthening self as represented by the plastic circle of self in their hands.

You can introduce **Handout 1: Relationship Circles** (p. 7) using the following introductory script.

Psychoeducation Script
Introduction to Relationship Circles

A practical way to understand codependency is "loss of self in someone else." As you are learning, when we are too externally focused, we lose our connection with self. One way to understand this loss of self is through a visual tool called relationship circles, which is illustrated in this handout. Let's take a look at it now.

After studying the handout with its accompanying script, you can use **Client Worksheet 3: Relationship Circles** to help your client examine their relationship style (or styles).

Relationship Circles

Study

Have you ever had the experience of losing your self in someone else? If so, what did that feel like to you? What were your experiences? What did you do?

_____

_____

_____

_____

To further understand your experience of loss of self, let's work with **Handout 1: Relationship Circles**. Carefully read through the descriptions of each type of relationship illustrated by the relationship circles.

Now, think of a relationship in which you lost your healthy connection with your self. Which relationship style describes your relationship with that person?

_____

_____

Let's look at what may be some of _your part_ in the relationship style you have identified. Your part is where you have power to learn, grow, and change.

- If you have an **enmeshed relationship**, do you have trouble leaving the other person alone? Does the other person make it hard for you to separate from them and be your own person?

_____

_____

- If you have an **alienated relationship,** do you avoid the other person, stay away, or try not to engage them any more than necessary?

_____

_____

- If you have a **healthy relationship**, are you able to speak your truth to this person, express your needs, and offer the same to them? Are you able to identify when you may need space, and can you honor when they need space from you?

_____

_____

Self-Reflection

Are you noticing anything about your self and how you tend to interact in your relationships?

_____

_____

Which relationship style would you prefer for your self?

_____

_____

Are there any changes in you that you might want to make in order to have the relationship style you prefer?

_____

_____

Notes to Self

_____

_____

_____

_____

Strategy 22

Use the **balance scale** diagram.

Handout 6: Self/Other Balance Scale (p. 34) is a clear, simple image to help assess where your client is placing their focus and resources. It can also be a solid tool for psychoeducation. If you have not already used this handout for assessment, offer it to your client for self-study. Work through the handout together, explaining how the scale shows the balance between self and other, between internal and external focus. Help them examine not only their feelings, needs, and wants but also the focus they bring to therapy. Who are they there to help: their self, another person, both? No judgment is called for. The goal is simply for both of you to get a feel for their level of self-connection early in their therapy work.

Strategy 23

Use the **continuum** diagram.

You were introduced to the continuum in **strategy 6** (p. 11). Now it's time to use it as a handout with your client. Revisit **Handout 4: Assessing for Behaviors Associated with Codependency** (p. 29) and ask your client to identify the top behaviors they engage in. Then, using **Handout 2: Codependency Behaviors Continuum** (p. 12), have them identify the extent to which they engage in those behaviors and the adjustments they want to make for self-recovery. The continuum teaches that there is nothing wrong with most behaviors associated with codependency. We can just carry them too far, which brings consequences for self and others.

Here is a case example to share with your client as you teach them about the continuum. Let's return to Cynthia, the 50-year-old mother whose adult daughter relapses from her alcohol recovery and habitually asks for help, often in the form of money.

Psychoeducation Script
Cynthia and the Continuum

Let's look at codependent behaviors on a continuum. This is an important visual tool that acknowledges that most behaviors associated with codependency are not unhealthy in and of themselves. You can just carry them too far and lose your self in others. Rather than waiting until you have gone too far, you can learn to regulate your self along this continuum. Self-regulation is an important part of self-recovery.

The following is a case example to help you understand how to use this continuum.

Cynthia's adult daughter, Jenna, has asked her mother for $300 to pay for her auto insurance for this month. This is a big ask for Cynthia. Jenna has been living with her mom, not paying rent, working retail part-time, and alternately relapsing from and recommitting to treatment for alcoholism. Given that Jenna has few expenses, Cynthia has no idea where Jenna spends her money; she tries to stay out of Jenna's business as best she can. She does not even know if Jenna really needs this money, but she worries that not giving it to her may cause Jenna to relapse.

Now let's use the continuum to study Cynthia's behavior of giving money.

At the "okay" end of the continuum, Cynthia keeps a centered connection with self as she considers giving money to Jenna. Cynthia knows she can give $100 to Jenna without causing herself any financial problems. Her giving has no strings attached; she is not hoping that Jenna will be grateful and do something to please her or give her something in return. Cynthia is clear on why she is giving and is glad that she can do so freely. She has a solid connection with her money, her decision, and her self.

If Cynthia considers providing more money to Jenna, this may be the beginning of her movement along the continuum toward "too far." Knowing that $100 is not all Jenna needs to pay her auto insurance, Cynthia decides to take an additional $200 out of her vacation savings account to give to Jenna. She would rather Jenna have the money than for her to stay an extra day or two on vacation. She is hopeful that if she gives Jenna the full amount she requested, Jenna will appreciate her generosity, do more things around the house, and work on her recovery.

Cynthia is moving toward too far as she loses track of her original decision to give $100, which felt right to her. She is also losing track of self by creating an unspoken transaction that expects Jenna to do more as a result of Cynthia's generosity. Unaware that this expectation is a way to try to manage and control Jenna, Cynthia will likely focus even more on Jenna's behaviors, hoping for her gratitude, help at home, and progress in her recovery. This unspoken "deal" can be a codependent tangle for both.

Movement on this continuum can be tricky; it requires awareness and discernment as a person makes decisions to extend their codependent behaviors. While there are no rules about offering more, as a person chooses to engage further in behaviors associated with codependency, it is important for them to be aware of self: their motivations, resources, hopes, and dreams. Cynthia would do well to check in with these aspects of self before giving that full $300 to Jenna. There are no right answers; the answers that promote growth are within Cynthia. By considering her self to the same extent that she considers Jenna, Cynthia is more likely to figure out what she can honestly offer without expectations and resentments.

The Continuum

Study

What do you think of this idea of looking at your behaviors on this continuum from *okay* to *too far*? Do you believe you can engage in a particular behavior from a lesser to a greater degree?

_____

_____

_____

_____

Self-Reflection

Identify one of your behaviors associated with codependency that you want to consider on the continuum. With your behavior in mind, walk through the following questions:

What behavior are you examining now? Simply naming it is helpful for promoting awareness and deeper consideration.

_____

_____

How do you feel when you engage in this behavior?

_____

_____

What might cause you to do more of this behavior? For what reasons might you start moving from okay toward too far?

_____

_____

Do you ever carry this behavior too far?

_____

_____

Would you like to modify or change this behavior?

_____

_____

There are no right or wrong answers to these questions. At this point in your work, the lesson is to become more aware of your behaviors, reasons, choices, and actions that may lead you too far.

Notes to Self

_____

_____

_____

_____

Strategy 24

Invite the client's shift to an aware and responsive **internal focus**.

Embedded within all this early psychoeducation is an invitation to our clients to increase their internal awareness and responsiveness. Each of the previous worksheets points the client in this important direction of internal focus. Very soon we will enter Part III: Self-Recovery Treatment. As we do so, let's clarify the value of this shift to an internal focus a bit more and extend the invitation by suggesting some safe, gentle actionable assignments to help them experience the beginnings of this shift.

Psychoeducation Script
The Importance of Internal Focus in Self-Recovery

As you are learning, codependency is about not being able to balance your focus on others with a healthy focus on self. When you came here for therapy, you probably did not know we would be looking at this underlying dynamic of self/other. You came with concerns about your anxiety, your depression, your relationships. Please know that we are working on those things through this self-recovery work. You can learn ways to manage anxiety, decrease depression, and communicate better with others. But if you don't also treat this loss-of-self-in-others way of being, you will still be vulnerable to health and relationship problems. This is because underfunctioning on your own behalf leads you to:

- Neglect your self, including your health, money, work, and friendships

- Fail to consider your self in important decisions and planning

- Develop physical or psychological problems

- Do things that are inconsistent with your values

- Put your self in vulnerable positions

Learning to focus on self in healthy, balanced ways opens the door to codependency recovery. You can then start functioning more kindly and effectively on your own behalf. In so doing, you not only prevent this list of problems, but you grow into greater health.

Making this shift from a dominant external focus to an aware, responsive internal focus takes commitment, time, and energy. I believe you can make this important fundamental change, and I'm ready to help as you do this for you!

To extend this invitation further, offer **Client Worksheet 5: Shifting to an Aware and Responsive Internal Focus**, which suggests actionable assignments that can help them experience the beginning of this shift.

Shifting to an Aware and Responsive Internal Focus

This Week

Think about the behaviors associated with codependency that you have identified as true for you. (You can refer back to **Handout 7: Assessing for Overfunctioning for Others/Underfunctioning for Self** as needed.) Pick two of your behaviors—including one example of overfunctioning for others and one example of underfunctioning for self—and watch for them this week as you live your life. Make some notes about at least one interaction for each of those behaviors. Just notice what you thought, felt, and did in that moment. No judgment—just notice your self.

_____

_____

_____

_____

_____

_____

_____

_____

_____

_____

_____

_____

Notes to Self

_____

_____

_____

_____

Insights and Intentions

Consider the strategies introduced in this chapter:

19. **Educate** about external versus internal focus.

20. **Illustrate** codependent dynamics using visual tools.

21. Use the **relationship circles** diagram.

22. Use the **balance scale** diagram.

23. Use the **continuum** diagram.

24. **Invite** the client's shift to an aware and responsive **internal focus**.

What have you learned in this chapter about helpful early psychoeducation about codependency?

_____

_____

_____

Which handouts or worksheets in this chapter seem particularly useful in your work with codependent clients?

_____

_____

_____

Have you had any realizations about your self?

_____

_____

_____

Are there handouts or worksheets from this chapter that you might intentionally bring to your practice or into your own life?

_____

_____

_____

CHAPTER 5

Important Basics for a Therapeutic Relationship with a Codependent Client

As clinicians, we are a frontline person in our client's life. We have the opportunity to make their relationship with us different from the ways they usually relate to others. We don't want to encourage their people-pleasing, conflict-avoiding tendencies. Nor do we want to struggle with them over control. Instead, we want to give them space and confidence to explore self and honor what is true for them. In this chapter, I will be highlighting specific clinician strategies that will help you guide your client in learning to trust, listen, and respond to self.

Strategy 25

Establish **mutuality** in therapeutic work.

Mutuality in our clinical work is foundational to self-recovery. The research of Bacon and Conway (2023) emphasizes the importance of fostering a codependent client's autonomy and attunement to self. Mutuality supports both these goals. Simply put, here's how it looks:

- You, the therapist, bring your knowledge and clinical experience to your work with your client.

- Your client brings who they are to the sessions as well as changes they are seeking for self.

- You work together to achieve *their* goals.

While this likely sounds obvious, clinicians sometimes lose track of the mutual process, feeling more than our fair share of responsibility for our client's work. We get attached to ideas of what they should and should not be doing, find ourselves frustrated with the choices our client is making, or inadvertently convey that they are wrong and we are right.

This is why it is best to be mindful as we go, aware not only of our client but of our self in the room, in the conversation, in our own motivations and intentions. Our own self-awareness is essential to sustaining the mutual curiosity and exploration we want to share with our clients.

Strategy 26

Encourage client **self-empowerment**.

As with healthy parenting, we want our therapeutic relationship with our client to lead them to a confident, autonomous life of their own. For this reason, it is essential to establish safety, good listening, understanding, and empathy early in our work with codependent clients.

As we begin building our relationship with a codependent client, we want to listen deeply and accurately so that the client feels heard by us. Over time, this will train them to hear themselves in kind and open ways and respond to what they hear within.

We also want to empower them. This involves gentle awareness of clients leaning in our direction when we can help them find what they seek within. We notice when they ask us what they "should" do or if it is "okay" that they feel a particular way. Early on, we may provide answers to some of these questions, but our goal is for them to know and trust their own decisions and feelings. We recognize when we are making direct statements or suggestions when mutual curiosity and exploring would be more self-empowering for our client. This clinical awareness is a gentle, back-and-forth process wherein the client feels heard by their therapist and also encouraged to go within and find their answers, a process fostering both the client-therapist relationship and the client's relationship-with-self.

There are specific moments and interventions within the therapy hour that can encourage self-empowerment. **Clinical Tip Sheet 1: Fostering Self-Empowerment Leads to Autonomy** lists some of those opportunities and therapeutic responses. Clinical themes include validation, invitations to self-reflect and express, and creation of self-assignments. Each tip invites your client to tune in to self and notice what is going on within.

Fostering Self-Empowerment
Leads to Client Autonomy

- Validate the client's choice to enter counseling.

- Validate the client's feelings, thoughts, and experiences.

- Have the client:

  - Self-reflect in verbal or written form

  - Assert their ideas, desires, and preferences

  - Make their own appointments related to their mental health care (including medical, psychiatric, or psychological testing and any other health-related services) once you have offered them referral names and contact information

  - Take their own notes in session

  - Take the lead on topics and ideas for discussion

  - Assign their own homework ("self-assignment")

- Use/reflect the client's words back to them.

- When they are storytelling, ask, "How does that affect you?"

- When we are not clear why they are describing something to us, ask, "Why is this important to you?"

- When we hear what they are saying, and there are several directions we could respond, ask, "What do you want from me in this moment/on that topic?"

Strategy 27

Foster the client's internal focus.

How do we help our clients with codependency increase their internal focus? Simply pointing it out to them likely won't make a significant change. Helping them understand in detail what this shift to an internal focus looks like, how this shift would help them, and ways to connect with self are essential threads in their tapestry of self.

Handout 9: Four Areas of Self (p. 53) can help foster internal focus. Use this illustration to remind your client of their four areas of self. Help them understand that each area is distinct and merits awareness and responsiveness, but emphasize that the areas overlap—responding to emotions can help the body, quieting thoughts may allow them to access spiritual sources beyond self, and so forth.

Helping your client access self is another way to foster internal focus. There are many reasons a client may have trouble accessing self, from the ego defense mechanisms articulated by Freud to the protective parts described in internal family systems, from common habits like obsessive thinking, compulsive behaviors, and addictions to everyday distractions like daily to-do lists, unrealistic expectations, and other-centeredness. Self-protection is common and necessary for many, but that protection can keep us from accessing the wisdom and strength within our self.

Helping your client access self should be a respectful, client-led process that simultaneously honors this need to protect self and invites increased internal focus. **Clinical Tip Sheet 2: Helping Clients Access Self** provides ideas and examples to guide you during sessions when opportunities appear to help your client access self.

Helping Clients Access Self

Helping our clients access self is essential to increasing their internal focus, making it a primary goal of codependency treatment. The following are a few suggestions for helping your client access self as they engage in self-recovery:

- Create internal space for your client.

  - Work at your client's pace. This may take time.

  - Bring flexibility to your sessions and the conversations within it.

  - Be nonjudgmental, accepting that the client is doing the best they can.

  - Bring patience, openness, and curiosity.

  - Laugh together.

  - Let them know you are glad to be with them.

  - Ask them what is important for them to talk about and how they wish to use their therapy time.

- Invite self-reflection.

  - Have the client check in periodically with their four areas of self.

  - Invite them to share with you whatever they may find within those four areas of self or anything else that may be coming up for them.

  - Offer self-reflective exercises (verbal or written), then ask:

    » "What does that mean to you?"

    » "What are your thoughts about that?"

    » "How would that be helpful to you?"

  - Use/reflect their words back to them.

    » "You said that was 'terrible' for you. Can you say more about that?"

    » "You said 'It is hard to be hopeful.' Can you say more about that?"

- Redirect to self.

  - When the client is telling stories about other people or situations in which they were not directly involved, ask:

    » "How does that affect you?"

    » "Why is this important to you?"

    » "What do you want from me in this moment/on that topic?"

- Use the visual tools (relationship circles, the balance scale, and the continuum) to help your client bring self into clear, accurate focus.

    » "Use these circles to show me how you interact with your partner."

    » "How does your balance scale of self/other look to you?"

    » "Where on this continuum do your codependent behaviors fall? In which direction are they moving?"

Strategy 28

Join the client at **their stage of change**.

Not only do we want to move in the same direction as our client, but we also want to move at their pace, supporting them as they venture further into their internal domains. Knowing the stages of change can help us get in synch (Prochaska & DiClemente, 1983). The stages of change provide markers of where your client is in their process of change, helping you make clinical sense of your client's pace and energy, which may range from reticent and cautious to clear, committed, and ready.

With treating codependency in particular, meeting the client where they are is a strong strategy for fostering their increased access to and comfort with internal awareness. After all, change is a process that involves multiple steps and stages. Successful work happens when their therapy goals are aligned with where they are in their change process instead of suggesting or encouraging things they are not yet ready for and letting your desire to hurry up and make things better for them take hold.

Clinical Tip Sheet 3: Stages of Changes and Codependency provides you with a description of each stage (from Prochaska & DiClemente, 1983), as well as clinical examples of ways codependent clients may present when they are in that stage of change.

Stages of Change and Codependency*

PRECONTEMPLATION

The client has no awareness that a problem exists.

For example:

- The client does not see that the way someone is treating them is problematic.

- They believe they are the problem.

- They are not aware of the importance of boundaries.

- They are not aware of their other-centeredness. They have never thought in this way before.

- They do not connect their sleep and appetite problems with their relationship entanglements.

CONTEMPLATION

The client is aware there is a problem. They are willing to consider making a change but not immediately.

For example:

- The client becomes aware that they do not like the way someone is treating them. They start to see that what they are doing does not merit the ways they are being treated by this other person.

- The client starts understanding healthy boundaries.

- They realize how little they consider themselves in their relationships.

- They start to connect their physical and emotional problems with their out-of-balance relationships with others.

PREPARATION

The client is ready to make a change in the near future. They believe the change will be good for them and that they can make the change. They learn new skills, gather social support, and prepare for obstacles.

For example:

- The client learns how to speak up for self.

- The client learns how to set healthy boundaries with self and with others.

- The client increases their awareness of their body, mind, emotions, and spirit.

- The client actively uses the self/other balance scale to be more aware of their other-centeredness.

---

* Based on the stages of change identified by Prochaska and DiClemente (1983).

ACTION

The client is practicing new behaviors. The client believes in their ability to change even when they run into obstacles or experience loss and grief.

For example:

- Before setting a boundary, the client takes time for self and considers all four areas of self and then formulates their "I" statement.

- The client practices using "I" statements to express self to others.

- The client makes sure to do something each day for self.

- The client is putting self into the formula of their life in a conscious, intentional way.

MAINTENANCE

The client continues to make desired changes. New behaviors and patterns replace old ones. These changes are supported and maintained by social support as well as internal rewards such as feeling happier, more peaceful, and less conflicted.

For example:

- The client uses therapy time to define and rehearse "I" statements.

- The client lets a friend know when they are going to speak up at home and makes arrangements to talk with their friend afterward.

- The client is journaling to increase self-awareness and grounding.

- The client learns to notice when to stop self as they are drawn into an entangled interaction.

RELAPSE

The client reacts to people or situations with their old behaviors and patterns. They recognize the thoughts and feelings they previously experienced and explore what triggered them to react in these former ways. The client restores their progress by noticing these things, reconnecting to their motivation to change, and fortifying their coping strategies.

For example:

- The client recognizes that they were tired when they relapsed and should have just gone to bed instead of engaging in an upsetting conversation.

- The client's anxiety was strong and they made an emotional decision to give more to someone else that what was needed.

- The client's desire to please someone else over their own needs caused them regret the next day.

- The client trusts that you, the therapist, will be nonjudgmental about their relapse and continue to support them as they resume action and maintenance.

Strategy 29

Inventory the essential **ingredients of change** together.

When we cook something, we study the list of ingredients. We also look at the ingredients of products we purchase and medications we take. Knowing what the substance is composed of informs our choices and actions. So it is with ingredients of change.

Over the years of my self-recovery work, I have developed a list of 10 ingredients needed for change (Johnston, 2020):

1. Awareness

2. Willingness

3. Intentionality

4. Self-education

5. Skill-building

6. Self-regard

7. Noticing self in the moment

8. Intervening on our own behalf

9. Spirituality

10. Letting go

Each of these ingredients will be incorporated into the self-recovery work that follows. For now, making the important shift from external focus to internal focus requires the top three ingredients of change in this order:

1. **Awareness:** Awareness is everything. If we are not aware of our self, we cannot know what we can change to improve our lives. Self-recovery brings many things into awareness, including our body, behaviors, language, and moods. Awareness opens the door to what we want to change, then supports and guides us as we make those changes moment by moment.

2. **Willingness:** Willingness is as essential to change as awareness is. We can become aware of our self and the changes we want to make yet lack willingness to do what it takes to make those changes. Fears, resistance, and self-protection may present themselves, inviting deeper work. Willingness to work with these important issues and parts then becomes the focus. *What am I willing to do? What am I willing to explore? Let go of? Try?* Any answer is fine.

3. **Intentionality:** Change can happen when we are aware and willing and we add intention. Intentionality means that we consciously speak, act, and make choices consistent with what we want to change in our self and our lives. We remember what we want for self and find ways to make our new goals and behaviors happen.

When your client is stuck in a stage of change or has relapsed, a look at these three ingredients of change may point the way to helpful clinical work: Are they **aware**? Are they **willing**? What are they ready to **intentionally** do for self-recovery?

Strategy 30

Address any **countertransference** and **codependency in self**.

As we establish a therapeutic relationship with clients with codependency, it is important to notice, acknowledge, and respond to whatever personal challenges may be coming up for us as clinicians.

In part, we are talking about *countertransference*. Countertransference is when the therapist's emotional reactions to the client or the therapist's own life experiences interfere with their ability to be objective, patient, and balanced in their engagement with their client. "Balanced" means not becoming overly friendly or overly disapproving of the client. The therapist must be able to listen to and respond to their client without reacting from their own unattended feelings, thoughts, and fears.

We are also talking about the possibility of codependency within the therapist. If present, this tendency can surface in sessions and interfere with the client's progress toward developing their relationship-with-self. Every clinician would do well to explore the possibility of having codependent features in themselves.

Let's look at these important clinical dynamics in more detail.

Countertransference

We may believe that we are neutral listeners—and often, we are—but sometimes we are triggered by things our codependent clients say or do. Successful treatment of codependency requires becoming aware of your emotional reactions to your clients and what you do with those emotions. When you are with your client, notice your reactions and identify the feelings you are experiencing. Despite our training and our good intentions, we can experience an assortment of feelings and impulses in reaction to a codependent client. Here are some of the possibilities:

- Care
- Concern
- Compassion
- Affection
- Admiration
- Hopes for them
- Plans for them
- Wishes for them

- Desire to fix things for them

- Judgment

- Frustration

- Discouragement

- Impatience

- Insistence

- Impulse to force them to do something

- Problem-solving for them

- Confusion

- Hopelessness

As you see from this list, our emotions can go in several directions—supportive and critical, patient and impatient, hopeful and frustrated. Our emotions can prompt us to say and do things in our therapy work that we would not say or do if we were aware of self and aware of the effects our words and actions have on the therapeutic relationship. With codependent clients in particular, our unprocessed emotions may make it more difficult for them to attend to their core tasks of keeping the focus on self and fostering their relationship-with-self.

Knowing that codependent clients are prone to people-pleasing and conflict avoidance, we want to make sure we are not creating a dynamic where they feel the need to please us. Knowing that codependent clients may want and need control, we don't want to fight with them. We want to encourage them to think and act on their own behalf, even if that means they take two steps forward and one step back. We create this space for our client's growth by managing the emotions, beliefs, and actions arising within us.

With your increased awareness of your reactions, take responsibility for your feelings so you don't act them out or impose them on your client. Notice them, breathe with them, and listen to them in that moment. Later, process your feelings outside of the therapy session, perhaps through your own therapy, journaling, movement, or mindfulness practices. Create space to hear, feel, and understand your self. Seek supervision, consultation, or further clinical training. On occasion, you may find it necessary to refer your client to another therapist if your countertransference is dominant and persistent.

Codependency

It is equally important to notice if you have codependent tendencies showing up in your work with a client. I am not suggesting that all therapists have codependent tendencies, merely that it is important to assess ourselves for them. We are, after all, professional helpers. Something within us makes us want to help, fix, and problem-solve. What we don't want to do is carry those behaviors too far and step into the self of the client, influencing them with our feelings and thoughts rather than fostering their own.

Our codependency can be the source of some of our countertransference. Our desires to help and fix can entangle us with our client. When we are offering so much to our client and they are not growing in the direction or at the pace we hoped, we may likely experience some of the emotions on the countertransference list. When we are aware of and take care of our codependent behaviors, we will have less countertransference and naturally create more space for our client's growth.

Your awareness of your codependency is the starting point for taking responsibility for it. Hopefully you have already learned a great deal about codependency in this workbook. Though it is written for your use with clients, it is also material for you to bring into your personal awareness and action, if you choose.

Here are a few things to especially take note of for self:

- Do I have a strong external focus?

- Do I look to others for approval and guidance rather than accessing those things in myself?

- Do I operate from the expectations of others without tuning into my self?

- Which codependent behaviors do I engage in?

- Do I carry those behaviors too far?

- Am I aware of those behaviors when they are happening and can I stop myself?

- Am I aware of when my self/other balance is off? Do I know how to correct it?

- Do I overfunction for others? If so, in what ways?

- Do I underfunction for myself? If so, in what ways?

- How do I feel about the things I am bringing into my awareness?

- Are there any changes I would like to make on my own behalf?

If you find that codependency resonates for you, be especially mindful of treatment suggestions that appeal to you as you study the four elements of self-recovery in part III.

Insights and Intentions

Consider the strategies introduced in this chapter:

25. Establish **mutuality** in therapeutic work.

26. Encourage client **self-empowerment**.

27. **Foster** the client's internal focus.

28. Join the client at **their stage of change**.

29. Inventory the essential **ingredients of change** together.

30. Address any **countertransference** and **codependency** in self.

What have you learned in this chapter about important basics for establishing a therapeutic relationship with a codependent client?

_____

_____

_____

Which strategies in this chapter seem particularly useful in your work with codependent clients?

_____

_____

_____

Have you had any realizations about your self?

_____

_____

_____

Are there strategies from this chapter that you might intentionally bring to your practice or into your own life?

_____

_____

_____

Part III

Treatment: The Four Interlocking Elements of Self-Recovery

You have learned to conceptualize and assess for codependency. You have acquired a number of visual tools and client worksheets to help you set the stage for change. All of this early work is itself treatment for codependency. Helping your client become aware of their dominant other-centeredness and its relationship to their presenting problems is foundational to their healing. Moreover, through mutual assessment and psychoeducation, you have invited them to begin to turn in safe, manageable ways toward self. Here in part III, you will learn many treatment strategies for helping your client develop the clear and secure relationship-with-self that we have been telling them is possible.

Years ago as I introduced the strategy of "detaching" to a client, she said, "I understand what you mean, Nancy, but how do I do that?" A great question—*how* do we detach? That question prompted my subsequent work on relationship entanglements and brings me here now with treatment ideas for your clients, who will be wondering: How do I detach? How do I not react? How do I set boundaries? How do I consider my self? What do I do with my guilt and anxiety?

In recent years, my self-recovery treatment model took solid form as a result of an interaction with a client who, in her anger with her partner, said regrettable things in unkind ways. As I listened to her story, I was aware of her loss of self in the interaction, and it became clear to me how much our health depends on recovering self—both restoring our connection with self in the moment and bringing health and healing to self over time. Let's look at each of these meanings of self-recovery.

First, self-recovery means literally restoring your connection with you when you are over-focused on someone else. As we go through life with a dominant external focus (for whatever helpful, protective, or obsessive reasons), it is easy to lose our connection with self. When we lose this connection, we act in regrettable ways. We say things we don't mean, deny our true feelings, and abandon our self.

There are a number of both internal and external experiences that interrupt our connection with self. Here are some examples shared by clients with codependent features:

- The person is not listening to me.

- I want to help and they won't let me.

- I want to please them.

- I want their approval.

- I am afraid they will leave me.

- I know I am right.

- I am afraid the other person will get in trouble.

- I am trying to guess what they are thinking and what they want.

- I am trying to get the other person to do something.

- I am generally anxious and try to find my stability through others.

- I want to know what others think of me so I know who I am.

These internal and external experiences are powerful challenges to self-recovery. That's why this part of the workbook includes in-depth strategies for helping your clients keep and foster their internal connections, especially when they are triggered by strong emotions and long-standing relational patterns.

Self-recovery also means caring for self in restorative and healing ways. Maybe your client had a healthy, balanced connection with self prior to specific life events. You can help them process their disconnections from self and then reconnect with the strengths and centeredness they used to have. In other cases, your client may never have known this type of healthy connection with self. With these clients, the therapy process helps them learn how to connect with and foster self so they can enjoy physical and emotional health.

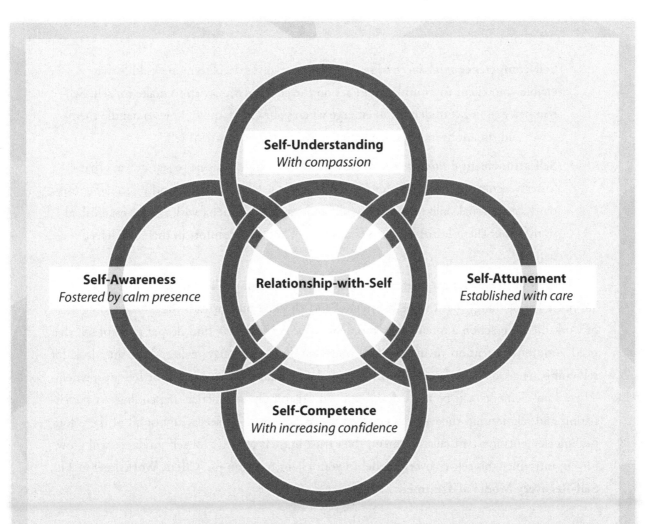

The self-recovery model involves four elements: self-understanding, self-awareness, self-competence, and self-attunement. The following image, which is also shown in **Handout 10: The Four Elements of Self-Recovery**, illustrates the interlocking nature of these four elements, with the relationship-with-self embraced in the center.

The details of each of these elements will be presented in the next four chapters, but here is a brief overview:

- **Self-understanding *with compassion*** involves looking at individuation, family of origin roles and rules, attachment styles, and trauma history. Self-understanding is about developing a compassionate awareness of individual tendencies, experiences, and parts of self that increase vulnerability to loss of self.

- **Self-awareness *fostered by calm presence*** enables your client to think, say, or act differently than they usually do. Awareness of self in the moment—body, mind, emotions, and spirit—gives them opportunities to respond kindly and effectively on their own behalf and to break out of their habitual patterns of reacting. In short, it opens the door to change.

- **Self-competence *with increasing confidence*** involves developing new skills that enable your client to formulate and act on the changes they wish to make for self. Self-competence and confidence can emerge when your client knows how to handle themselves and situations in ways that are effective and considerate of self.

- **Self-attunement *established with care*** means learning to attune to self in ways that foster a secure attachment with self. This involves listening and responding to self consistently. Additional skills for accessing self and staying in contact with self are established so that your client learns they can count on self and find comfort in their safe haven within.

These four interlocking elements of self-recovery are intentionally illustrated in a circle. They are not a list of things that can be completed and checked off. Instead, they are ongoing areas of work that interact on a moment-by-moment basis. A client may find deeper parts of self that need additional attention to increase self-understanding, they may realize skills they lack for self-competence, or they may have difficulty with cultivating self-awareness or self-attunement. These four elements will be needed and applied organically in practice, depending on the situation and relationship the client is engaged in. As they learn to access any or all of these four healing elements in a particular moment, their trust in their capacity for self-guidance will grow.

To introduce this self-recovery model to your client, you can use **Client Worksheet 6: The Self-Recovery Model of Treatment**.

The Four Elements of Self-Recovery

Self-Understanding
With compassion

Self-Awareness
Fostered by calm presence

Relationship-with-Self

Self-Attunement
Established with care

Self-Competence
With increasing confidence

The Self-Recovery Model of Treatment

Study

It's time to start learning things that will help you develop your relationship-with-self.

Handout 10: The Four Elements of Self-Recovery illustrates the self-recovery model we will be using. Self-recovery involves four elements of self-growth:

- Self-understanding
- Self-awareness
- Self-competence
- Self-attunement

Looking at the handout, notice the four interlocking rings that represent these healing elements. Also notice the center circle held within the four rings of self-development. This center circle represents the relationship-with-self you are developing.

The four elements are not a list that you can complete and check off. Instead, they are ongoing areas of work that interact on a moment-by-moment basis.

You can think of this image as a road sign, a logo, a map, a touchstone. It illustrates the interconnection of the work you will be doing. It can be a reminder of your goals, intentions, and ways to get where you want to be. It is an image to hold in your mind and heart as you move forward.

Self-Reflection

Let's take an introductory look at each of these four healing elements.

1) Self-Understanding

Self-understanding involves learning more about you. This includes understanding your basic nature and tendencies, your family history and experiences, and the influences of the worlds you live in. The more you understand about your self, the more you can appreciate why you have trouble keeping the focus on your self, and the more you will notice your disconnection from self when it happens.

What are your thoughts and feelings about increasing your self-understanding?

_____

_____

2) Self-Awareness

Self-awareness is foundational for change. Without your awareness, you will repeat your habitual, problematic patterns with self and others. You will react without thought. You will try to control what you cannot control. You will give beyond what you have to give. You will have no opportunity to say or do things differently. In short, you will lose connection with your self. Self-awareness, on the other hand, makes change possible and can become a lovely life companion, accompanying you wherever you may be.

What are your thoughts and feelings about increasing your self-awareness?

_____

_____

3) Self-Competence

Self-competence means learning new skills to help you connect with and respond to your self. You can't shift from being reactive to being responsive if you don't know how to calm your self. You can't say no if you don't know how. You can't take care of you if your guilt says you need to do more for others. Having more skills will help you strengthen your relationship-with-self and likely improve your confidence and comfort.

What are your thoughts and feelings about increasing your self-competence?

_____

_____

4) Self-Attunement

Self-attunement means that you create a sound, trustworthy connection with you. You know you will listen to your self and respond in kind and effective ways. You develop your internal focus and engage in daily practices that reassure you that you will be there for you. You feel grounded knowing that your relationship with you is secure.

What are your thoughts and feelings about increasing your self-attunement?

_____

_____

Notes to Self

_____

_____

_____

CHAPTER 6

Self-Understanding
with Compassion

Right from the beginning of my work with treating codependency, I recognized the need for self-understanding. Understanding self helps your client notice their tendencies to focus on others, know the source of those tendencies, and make conscious choices about doing their same old, same old or doing something different. Self-understanding also invites compassion and healing. As your client understands self better, they may find injuries and protective patterns that are sources of their dominant other-centeredness. Therapeutically addressing these sources is essential to self-recovery.

It is important that self-understanding be acquired with compassion. Our clients can be profoundly critical and harsh with self, judging or attacking their thoughts, feelings, and behaviors. No wonder they have not been willing or able to get to know self better. For this reason, as you work with clients on self-understanding, it is important to introduce, encourage, and facilitate compassion for self, no matter what they may come to understand about their developmental experiences and the choices they have made over their lifetime.

Self-understanding *with compassion* can be gained through your client's increased awareness of their basic nature and tendencies. It involves exploring the extent to which they were able to develop a sense of self separate from their family system, the roles and rules of their family of origin, their attachment styles, and their trauma history. Additionally, your client's understanding of the social, cultural, political, and religious worlds in which they were raised can help them make sense of their thoughts, feelings, and behaviors in the present. Through their compassionate awareness of these influences, they may better understand their tendencies to lose self in others.

Strategy 31

Introduce the **circles of influence on self-development.**

It's time to work with your client on **Handout 3: Circles of Influence on Self-Development** (p. 17). Perhaps you introduced your client to this handout during your intake interview or in early psychoeducation. Now we will dive into a careful study of each layer of influence. This illustration explains our individuality, reminding us that the influences we have each experienced come together in their own unique ways.

Study this handout with your client, spending time with the written descriptions of each layer. This image alone can help your client begin to get to know self in manageable and safe ways.

Strategy 32

Explore **individual influences**.

Our genetic influences definitely play a role in our formation of self. We know that many of our identifying traits are inherited, from our hair and eye color, height, and tendency (or not) toward baldness to our specific emotional states and personality characteristics. For clinicians, it has become standard to ask a client if there is a family history of any number of things, such as breast cancer and heart disease, depression and anxiety, bipolar disorders, and addiction. We do this because recognizing our basic nature helps us to understand our self. Examining the psychological traits and characteristics we carry allows us to figure out what we want to do with them. I am not saying that codependency is genetic. My clinical work has found, however, that some of us have basic natures that can lead to loss of self in others as our life experiences (i.e., our "nurture") interplay with our nature. In particular, there are a few core characteristics that specifically may contribute to the development of codependent tendencies.

A readiness to extend self to others is one such characteristic. This includes being kind, thoughtful, and considerate. It can manifest as generosity with time, resources, and heart. The person is giving and sensitive to the world around them, aware of the feelings and needs of others, and ready to respond to them. Their moods may be deeply affected by the moods and behaviors of others.

Another core characteristic of the codependent person is the ability to get things done. A person with these traits is often a hard worker and does things well. They are reliable, loyal, and dedicated— you can count on them.

Anxiety is often present in clients who struggle with codependency. Anxiety, in moderate doses, is important to our survival. However, in larger doses or when it is unneeded, anxiety can result in unnecessary worry, unhelpful actions, and exhaustion. Anxiety may present itself as a driver of a client's codependency in ways like the following:

- **Worry and difficulty controlling worry:** Worry is powerful and tenacious. It disturbs the psyche and the body. It can move a person into action and away from self. Difficulty controlling worry can be dominant in a codependent client and range from concerns that they disappointed someone to fears that this person will never speak to them again.

- **Obsessive thoughts:** You likely have experience with a client whose mind keeps going over and over the same thing, who seems highly resistant to getting off the track they are on. Even if a session seems to bring them some resolution of a topic, in short order their focus is back on that topic. With codependent clients, this focus is often on the person they are worried about or what they, the client, may have done wrong.

- **Compulsive behaviors:** As with obsessive thinking, compulsive behaviors are demanding and persistent. People with compulsive tendencies may have a strong need to have things a particular way and cannot let go of this need until it is satisfied. They may cling to order, rules, and lists. Conscious or unconscious, these behaviors help them manage anxiety. Specifically, a codependent client's need to control people and situations may help them, for a brief while, feel calmer and in control of their own life.

- **Addictions:** One of the criteria for addiction as defined in the *DSM-5* (APA, 2013) is unsuccessful efforts to control use of a substance. Process addictions, such as gambling, pornography, and relationships, can also be identified by loss of control over use. Addictions are compulsions carried to an extreme. With codependency, this is when a person's behaviors associated with codependency are driven by fears, obsessive worries, and out-of-control actions to the too far end of the continuum.

Remember, we are looking at these individual influences on self-development to help your client compassionately understand their traits and tendencies that may contribute to their codependent ways of being. Then, with this understanding, they can begin to learn how to embrace and parent their core features as part of their self-recovery process.

Individual Influences on Self-Development

Study

Take a moment to study **Handout 3: Circles of Influence on Self-Development**. Notice the three concentric circles that nest within each other. This is an image of you and the influences on who you are today. As you consider each layer, you will understand more about you.

Now let's study the center circle, **individual influences**. This is about your basic nature, your innate tendencies. Please bring nonjudgment to this self-exploration work. The intent is for you to become more aware, loving, and accepting of your basic nature and to learn to embrace and parent your qualities.

How would you describe your basic nature? Perhaps you have never thought about you in this way before—that's okay. The time has come to name some of your core characteristics. Examples may include being shy, energetic, risk-taking, sensitive, thoughtful, hopeful, helpful, conscientious, and so forth. See what words come to you that feel true to you.

_____

_____

Self-Reflection

We are now going to look at some core tendencies that may contribute to codependency. These tendencies are normal and can contribute to a good life, but if we carry them too far, they can cause us to lose our self in others. We can overfunction for others and underfunction for self. Consider if any of these natural traits may be true for you.

Do you readily extend your self to others? Do you naturally give your time and energy to help others? Do you like to help people solve their problems? Do you think of your self as a "fixer"?

_____

_____

Do you think of your self as thoughtful, considerate, or kind? Are you generous?

_____

_____

Do you work hard and do a good job usually? Are you reliable and loyal? Can people count on you?

_____

_____

Are you inclined to be anxious?

_____

_____

Are you a "worrier"? Do you worry too much of the time? Is it hard for you to control your worry?

_____

_____

Are your thoughts sometimes obsessive or difficult to stop?

_____

_____

Do you have any behaviors that feel compulsive to you, like you *must* do them?

_____

_____

Do you have a strong need to be in control of people and situations?

_____

_____

Now, look at the characteristics you have identified as true for you. Could some of those traits contribute to losing your self in others if they go too far? Which ones?

_____

_____

_____

_____

Notes to Self

_____

_____

_____

_____

Strategy 33

Explore **family influences**.

The second ring in the circle of influences on self-development is family. Family affects the individual in one way or another across the individual's lifetime. Family influences include the client's family of origin as well as their intergenerational family. As we join our clients in looking at their experiences with their parents, we acknowledge that their parents were directly affected by their own parents. Looking back at previous generations can bring understanding and compassion. It can also motivate change for self and generations to come.

In this section, we will be spending time with five important ways to understand self relative to family:

- Individuation and differentiation

- Family roles and rules

- Attachment styles

- Trauma history

- Parts of self

It is fascinating how each of these family influences can contribute to codependency. Losing self in others can be understood in profound ways as we look with our client at their formative experiences. The first two topics in the previous list come from family systems work. Studying them will help your client see the ways their family operated, perhaps unknowingly, in order to maintain the family system's status quo. Though some of the rules, roles, and norms of their family system may have been problematic, the overall intent was to stabilize the family whether it was dysfunctional or not. Change can be more threatening than sustaining what is known and familiar.

The second two topics, attachment styles and trauma history, focus specifically on the ways your client was treated as a child. You and your client will consider their attachment styles. You will also safely look at any neglect, abuse, and trauma they may have experienced and consider what is needed now for their healing from these experiences.

The final topic, parts of self, acknowledges the importance and usefulness of this treatment focus. Working with the self-recovery model, you will learn ways to help your client identify parts of self that have developed as a result of their formative experiences. You will learn how to help your client meet, greet, and work with their parts so they can access self more fully and build their relationship-with-self.

Family influences is a very big topic. Full-length books have been written and entire graduate school courses have been taught about each of these five ways we are impacted by our family. In this workbook, I will give you and your client enough information for a basic understanding of the topic and how it relates to codependency. Along the way, I will provide references if you wish to do more in-depth study of any of these areas of family influence.

Strategy 34

Consider **individuation and differentiation**.

Individuation means the extent of a person's ability to be an individual separate from their family system. This does not mean leaving one's family of origin but rather being able to both be with your family and be an individual within your family. This is healthy individuation, something that codependent clients may not have achieved.

To understand this more fully, let's look again at the work of Murray Bowen (1978), who developed the intergenerational family systems theory. Seeing the family as a system of interconnected parts, Bowen explains that the goal of these interrelated parts is to maintain the status quo of the family system regardless of how well that family system is functioning. Bowen specifically names anxiety as the primary emotion influencing the family system dynamics. To maintain the system's homeostasis, different members respond in different ways to the anxiety felt within the family system, but all share the goal of not rocking the family boat.

Gilbert (2004) describes Bowen's family system dynamics as *a fusion of selves* rather than members having individual selves, resulting in an emotional unit wherein any emotion that affects one member affects all. Fusion of selves can also be called *enmeshment*. In **Handout 1: Relationship Circles** (p. 7), the first set of circles reflects enmeshment. The two individuals have very little (if any) connection with self; the two circles eclipse each other. This is a *static system*, meaning that the individuals are stuck in relationship patterns that do not support individuation. Bacon and Conway (2022) maintain that codependency is an outward manifestation of enmeshment. They say enmeshment occurs because the individual was not encouraged to develop their autonomy, nor did they receive parental attunement. As a result, the codependent individual developed a focus on meeting the needs and demands of others.

A goal in Bowen's family systems work is for a person to successfully differentiate who they are from others in their family system. *Differentiation of self* is one of the eight concepts of Bowen theory (Kerr, 2019). A differentiated person remains calm and clearheaded in the face of conflict. They are able to make thoughtful decisions not clouded by emotion or relationship pressures. There is consistency between what they say and do. They are confident in their thinking and define self without being pushy or wishy-washy. Even in the presence of their own anxiety, a differentiated person is able to be around people important to them and not feel responsible for them or controlled by them. Their emotional regulation, confidence, and clarity support the shift from other-centeredness to a healthy regard for self. This is what self-recovery looks like.

Individuation Versus Enmeshment

Study

Let's look again at **Handout 1: Relationship Circles**. These circles can help you understand *individuation*.

The first set of circles in the handout illustrates *enmeshment*, which we are studying in particular here. Enmeshment is the opposite of individuation.

Individuation means how much you are able to be your own person with your own thoughts, feelings, and needs. It also includes how well you are able to express your self to others even when you feel nervous or are afraid the other person will not be pleased by what you have to say. Individuation means you have things you enjoy and, as we say, have your own life, even as you are in relationships with others.

Self-Reflection

Consider your family of origin and your relationships with your parents. To what extent have you been able to individuate from them? Have you been able to become your own person?

_____

_____

Were you encouraged to develop your own ideas and interests? Was it okay to express your feelings?

_____

_____

What were some of your challenges to individuating in the past? Do you have challenges now?

_____

_____

Here are some descriptions of a person who has individuated from their family of origin in healthy ways. Make some notes about how true each of these may be for you. An individuated person:

• Is able to be around family members without feeling unnecessarily responsible for them.

_____

_____

• Is able to be around family members without feeling controlled by them.

_____

_____

- Is able to think for self.

  _____

  _____

- Is able to express their own thoughts and feelings.

  _____

  _____

- Trusts their own judgment and is able to take action using that judgment.

  _____

  _____

- Takes responsibility for their own life.

  _____

  _____

What do you understand about your individuation? Where are you at today with establishing your own self?

_____

_____

_____

_____

_____

_____

_____

_____

Notes to Self

_____

_____

_____

_____

97

Strategy 35

Consider family **rules and roles**.

Family rules and roles are part of a family system. Rules and roles are established to maintain the status quo of the system, whatever that might look like. Often these rules and roles are not spoken, but everyone in the family system knows them.

Family Rules

Rules may be explicit or inferred through behaviors and responses in the family system. Family members know what is okay and not okay to say or do. Having your own opinion may not be allowed. Expressing your feelings may have no place. Speaking the truth may be forbidden.

In Claudia Black's seminal work, *It Will Never Happen to Me: Growing Up with Addiction as Youngsters, Adolescents, Adults* (1981/2020), she presents three primary rules active in a troubled family: don't talk, don't trust, and don't feel. A simple read of these family restrictions immediately shows us why someone in such a household is not likely to have a separate sense of self. Denial of speech, trust, and feelings shuts off access to self.

Don't talk means just that: don't talk about your concerns or feelings, don't talk about what is really going on, don't be honest. If you do talk, you will upset others, and you may feel guilty about speaking up. The don't talk rule causes a person to mistrust their own perceptions and increases their tolerance for unacceptable behaviors. The don't talk rule silences the family members and fosters a silent self.

Don't trust means that you cannot safely believe that a family member will be there for you. You cannot count on your parents to meet your physical and emotional needs. It is not safe to share your thoughts and feelings. The don't trust rule damages a person's ability to trust in other relationships over their lifetime. It also damages their ability to trust self.

Don't feel means it is not okay to recognize and experience your own feelings. To abide by this rule, the child learns to minimize or deny their own emotions in order to maintain the stability of the family system. The don't feel rule is problematic for the individual both as a child and as an adult. Not having familiarity with a wide range of emotions and knowledge of what to do with those feelings makes it very difficult to access self.

These three rules show us how a person may develop codependency and loss of self in others. Though the family system retains its status quo as a result of these rules, individuals within the system have been silenced. Their independent thoughts and feelings have no place. No one is interested. No one wants to hear about it. It is all too threatening to the family system. As a result, the person living by these rules becomes dominantly other-centered. Denial of self is required for survival of the family system. Rule-abiding keeps everything contained and predictable, which can feel "close enough" to safety and happiness.

Family Rules

Study

Claudia Black's book *It Will Never Happen to Me: Growing Up with Addiction as Youngsters, Adolescents, Adults* (1981/2020) offers plenty of solid information for helping people who grew up in troubled families.

Black teaches three family rules that are present in such dysfunctional families. Often these rules are not spoken, but everyone in the family system knows them because it's how they were raised from birth or what they've experienced since joining the family.

1. **Don't talk:** Don't talk about your feelings, your concerns, or what is really going on in the family. Don't be honest and certainly don't upset others. That will upset the whole family. Speaking up is not okay.

2. **Don't trust:** You can't count on your family members to take care of your physical and emotional needs or to be there for you when you need support or help. It is not safe to share your thoughts and feelings. To share self makes you vulnerable to unreliable and perhaps harmful family members.

3. **Don't feel:** It is not okay to recognize and experience your own emotions. This rule teaches you to minimize or deny your own feelings in order to maintain the stability of the family system. Because you silence your emotions, you don't learn to recognize normal, legitimate emotions, nor do you know how to handle them when you are aware of them.

Self-Reflection

Now that was a lot of information packed in three briefly described family rules. Take some time to absorb the rules, and then make some notes about your experiences growing up with each rule.

1. Don't talk: _____

   _____

   _____

2. Don't trust: _____

   _____

   _____

3. Don't feel: _____

   _____

   _____

How might these rules be influencing your life now?

_____

_____

_____

_____

_____

_____

Perhaps you experienced the opposites of these rules. If so, how have you benefited from family rules that encouraged your development of self?

_____

_____

_____

_____

_____

_____

Notes to Self

_____

_____

_____

_____

Family Roles

Family roles also help to maintain homeostasis. If one person is upset, someone else needs to be calm and helpful. If one person has caused trouble, someone else needs to make the family proud.

Most of the roles we took on in our family of origin were not conscious—they were not assigned to us, nor did we necessarily pick them. Instead, they naturally emerged from our nature and in response to the dynamics within our family system.

All the family roles served to protect and ensure the survival of each person and the family system. The problem comes when we are rigidly attached to our roles even when they no longer work for us as they did in our family of origin. Because we are not necessarily aware of our roles, we are often unaware of the ways they are with us today. Or we may be aware but have no idea how to act and think in new ways. We are locked into our familiar, habitual ways of being and have not learned to respond to situations by using our internal awareness and wisdom.

Discussing family roles with clients can shed light on their long-standing habits and patterns of relating. Your clients can learn to pay attention to self and the situation at hand so they can choose their response, rather than acting out old scripts written long ago for their roles at that time. This is what it means to foster self-understanding *with compassion* for the child who survived back then and the adult who wants to grow and thrive now.

Claudia Black's (1981/2020) family roles are described in **Handout 11: Family Roles**.

Family Roles

Looking at your role (or roles) in your family system can be informing. Each person in your family has their particular roles, which helps to keep the family's status quo, no matter how healthy or troubled that system might be. Studying these roles can help you see how your old roles may be playing out in unhelpful ways in your life today.

In *It Will Never Happen to Me* (1981/2020), Claudia Black identifies five roles within a troubled family system:

1. **The responsible child:** The responsible child steps in to maintain consistency and safety in their home. They can be counted on to take care of family members and details of family life.

2. **The adjuster:** The adjuster steps out of the way when conflict or disturbance occurs in the household. They prefer to avoid being directly involved in what is happening and simply adjust to it.

3. **The placater:** The placater is a pro at taking care of the emotional needs of family members. Very attuned to others, their role is to protect others from their fears, sadness, and guilt.

4. **The mascot:** The mascot is the entertainer, the comic, the quick wit who keeps the family laughing and seeming to be happy. Their humorous style distracts from the family's pain, and they receive positive attention for the relief this provides everyone in the family.

5. **The acting-out child:** This child acts out their upset feelings. They might do this through a variety of behaviors, including lying, cheating, and defying authority and rules. The problems they create distract from the deeper issues within a troubled family.

Family Roles

Study

Read **Handout 11: Family Roles**, studying the five family roles described by Claudia Black. Each role served an important purpose in your family system, and none of the roles is better than others.

Self-Reflection

What role (or roles) do you identify with?

_____

_____

_____

_____

What purpose did your role serve in your family system? What did it accomplish (such as keeping the peace, distracting from the family's problems, or helping others)?

_____

_____

_____

_____

Do you play the same role today in any way?

_____

_____

_____

_____

What are the benefits of playing the role now? What are the costs to you of playing the role now?

_____

_____

_____

_____

Do you feel like you have to play that same role or are you able to choose whether to play it depending on the situation?

_____

_____

_____

_____

Would you like to not always play the same role? What do you think would happen if you didn't?

_____

_____

_____

_____

You don't always have to play the same old role. Self-recovery will help you learn new ways of being so you don't always have to use your familiar, habitual scripts.

Notes to Self

_____

_____

_____

_____

Strategy 36

Consider **attachment styles**.

In 2009, I presented on codependency at a conference in North Carolina. A woman in the front row raised her hand and asked if the loss of self in someone else is related to attachment styles. What an excellent question! At that point, I was coming from the addiction recovery models of treatment and had woven mindfulness practices into that work; I had not yet begun to consider attachment theory as a direct influence on codependency. Her question opened me to incorporating this into my work.

Acknowledging the large amount of information available on attachment theory, let's take a brief look at the basics and begin to see how attachment styles can influence the development of codependency.

Attachment theory was developed by British psychiatrist John Bowlby (1988) in the 1950s and 60s. The basic tenets of attachment theory are that an infant has an innate need to develop a relationship with at least one primary caregiver for healthy social and emotional development, and the patterns established in this primary relationship carry into the child's future relationships. The primary determinant of attachment or caregiver bond is not food, but the responsiveness of the caregiver to the infant's signals for safety, security, and protection.

An infant becomes securely attached to a primary caregiver who is sensitive and responsive to their needs on a consistent basis. These qualities produce a warm and enjoyable relationship for both the child and caregiver and foster the child's mental health. These relational experiences create within the child an *internal working model*—that is, a system of thoughts, beliefs, memories, and expectations about self, others, and the world. Emotions and behaviors also become part of this internal working model. The model is created from not only the child's experiences but also the feelings they experienced as a result of how they were treated. If the primary caregiver offers safety and support, the child is likely to develop a positive image of self and their expectations of others. If, however, the child receives neglect or abuse, they are likely to develop a negative image of self and what they can expect from others.

In the 1960s and 70s, Mary Ainsworth, a developmental psychologist, and her colleague advanced the research on attachment theory by establishing the concept of the attachment figure as a "secure base" from which the child can explore the world. She also identified three attachment styles in infants: *secure*, *insecure avoidant*, and *insecure ambivalent/resistant* (Ainsworth & Bell, 1970; Ainsworth et al., 1979/2015).

We will study these styles more thoroughly in **Client Worksheet 11: Attachment Styles**; however, even a glance will help us understand why some people are more inclined to focus on others and to express their anxieties through this dominant other-centeredness. With either of the insecure attachment styles, the individual does not trust the person they are in a relationship with, so they hold on tight to them (insecure ambivalent/resistant) or are strongly independent against them (insecure avoidant). Because they do not experience their own worthiness and lovability, they overfunction to keep the person from leaving them, or else they fear intimacy and won't get close. An insecure attachment style contributes to an insecure sense of self and the loss of self in others.

Research in attachment theory continued with psychologist Mary Main, who identified a fourth attachment style: *disorganized* (Main & Solomon, 1986). A child with this attachment style has no coherent way of coping. Their behaviors reflect both a desire for their caregiver and fear of them, a mix of the ambivalent/resistant and avoidant characteristics. Trauma may well be a reason for this disorganized attachment style.

We will work more with attachment styles in the fourth self-recovery element: self-attunement. For now, use **client worksheet 11** to study Ainsworth's three attachment styles and help your client see what self-understanding *with compassion* they may gain. Here is a script to introduce the worksheet.

Psychoeducation Script
Attachment Styles

A psychiatrist named John Bowlby developed what is called attachment theory. He was interested in the relationship between an infant and their primary caregiver. Bowlby determined that a secure relationship was created when the caregiver was sensitive and responsive to the child on a consistent basis.

Mary Ainsworth, a psychologist, expanded Bowlby's work through research with children and their primary caregivers. She found three attachment styles: secure, insecure avoidant, and insecure ambivalent/resistant.

We all have basic needs for a secure relationship—that is, one in which we feel safe, confident, and protected. The attachment style we develop depends on how well these needs were fulfilled through how we were treated as children. If our parents or caregivers were attuned and responsive to us consistently, we likely have a secure attachment style. We knew we could count on our caregivers, and that helped us feel comfortable trusting other people throughout our lives, making us more likely to develop good relationships with others and with our selves.

However, if our parents were not attuned, responsive, and predictable in the ways they treated us, we likely developed an insecure attachment style (for good reason). With an insecure attachment style, we find it more difficult to trust and connect with other people and even with our selves.

Take a moment to think about this concept of attachment style. What are your thoughts and feelings about this idea? Do you have any questions for me about this material so far? When you are ready, we have a worksheet that will teach you more about the three attachment styles.

Attachment Styles

Study

Attachment styles are characterized by how you feel, what you think, and how you behave in relationship with important others. Attachment styles develop from our relationship with our primary caregiver in the first couple of years of our life. Read through the following descriptions of the three attachment styles. Take time to consider each one. Remember, you are working on self-understanding *with compassion*. This work can be exciting and challenging, enlightening and ultimately freeing.

1) Secure Attachment

The child has experienced their caregiver's sensitivity, warmth, and consistency and sees their caregiver as a secure base from which to explore their world. The child has developed an internal security that gives them confidence, comfort, and the ability to grow.

Have you developed a secure attachment style through your growth? To what extent do you identify with this description of a secure attachment?

_____

_____

_____

_____

2) Insecure Avoidant Attachment

The child with an insecure avoidant attachment style has experienced their caregiver as emotionally unavailable to them. The caregiver has not been able to validate and respond to the child's feelings and perhaps discouraged neediness and crying. Encouraged to be independent, a child with this style experiences no attachment and keeps their distance. Their sense of self is low.

Have you developed an insecure avoidant attachment style through your growth? To what extent do you identify with this attachment style?

_____

_____

_____

_____

3) Insecure Ambivalent/Resistant Attachment

A child with this attachment style has received inconsistent responses from their primary caregiver that ranged from appropriate to neglectful. Never knowing what to expect from their caregiver, the child feels anxious. They are preoccupied with their attachment figure but are unable to establish a secure, relationship with that person or with self.

Have you developed an insecure ambivalent/resistant attachment style through your growth? To what extent do you identify with this attachment style?

_____

_____

_____

_____

Self-Reflection

What are your thoughts about these attachment styles and your own experience?

_____

_____

_____

_____

How are you feeling about these attachment styles and your own experience?

_____

_____

_____

_____

Are you seeing any relationship between your attachment style and your tendencies to overfocus on others to the neglect of your self?

_____

_____

_____

_____

If you have an insecure attachment style, how does that show up in your relationships now? Are you holding on for fear of being left? Giving mixed messages about wanting to be close *and* wanting the person to go away? What is true for you?

_____

_____

_____

_____

Know that you can change your attachment style. The first step is becoming aware of your style. This awareness prepares you to learn and practice self-recovery strategies that can help you establish a secure relationship with your self, a relationship that offers the security you naturally seek and creates a foundation for healthy relationships with others.

Notes to Self

_____

_____

_____

_____

Strategy 37

Consider trauma history.

The family influences we have been studying—individuation versus fusion, family roles and rules, and attachment styles—all involve childhood experiences that were, too often, traumatic. In this strategy, I offer a reminder of the powerful role trauma plays in creating codependency. As with the other family influences, I will present important general information on this topic and offer references and resources for more in-depth study of trauma and healing.

Types of Trauma

Post-Traumatic Stress Disorder

A person with PTSD experienced, witnessed, or was repeatedly exposed to the aversive details of one or more events that involved actual or threatened death, serious injury, or a threat to the physical integrity of self or others. Within this experience, the person suffered intense fear, helplessness, or horror. As a result of these intense experiences, in order to protect self, the person develops distressing symptoms that involve re-experiencing the trauma or persistent avoidance of things that remind them of the trauma.

This has been our classic understanding of trauma. However, we have come to understand that trauma does not have to meet all the *DSM-5* criteria for PTSD to be an essential focus of treatment. Relational trauma and complex trauma must also be assessed for and treated for deep and full self-recovery to take place.

Relational Trauma

Relational trauma comes from the attachment wounds we studied in the previous strategy. When a child has not been responded to by their primary caregiver in sensitive, responsive, and consistent ways, they develop an insecure attachment style. Their insecurities can present with anxiety and preoccupation with their caregiver. They may be hypervigilant, scanning their environment for safety and security, or they may distance or remove themselves to protect against future disappointments and neglect.

These responses have neurobiological bases and effects. During the first 24 months of life, the child's nervous system is developing. Bonding and attachment are essential to healthy neurological development. We are wired for love and relationships. When a child has to protect themselves from harm, the energy they expend and the behavioral patterns they create for survival thwart their development of their true self and meaningful relationships (Ainsworth et al., 1979/2015; Lampis & Cataudella, 2019).

Complex Trauma

Complex trauma involves interpersonal traumatic stressors—that is, traumas caused by one person harming, violating, or exploiting another human being. Often, these traumatic experiences have been repetitive, prolonged, and perpetrated by primary caregivers during developmentally vulnerable times such as childhood and adolescence. Examples of such traumatic experiences include:

- Physical abuse

- Emotional abuse

- Sexual abuse

- Discrimination

- Humiliation

- Neglect

- Growing up in a household with:

  - Active addiction

  - Domestic violence

  - Mental illness

  - Incarceration or hospitalization of a family member

  - Absence of both parents

  - Poverty

The effects of complex trauma are numerous and profound. The individual may have trouble regulating their emotions, problems with attention, difficulty with intimacy, and an array of medical problems. They often suffer from deep hopelessness and helpless, a negative sense of self, and a battered identity. Rich information about treating complex trauma has been offered by therapists such as Arielle Schwartz (2016, 2021), Janina Fisher (2021, 2022), and Richard Schwartz and Martha Sweezy (2020).

Effects of Trauma

Neurobiology

Trauma causes an individual to be on high alert for cues of danger in order to protect self. When the person feels threatened, the amygdala (an "alarm" in the brain that responds to emotionally charged stimuli) signals the sympathetic nervous system (SNS) to release adrenaline, cortisol, and norepinephrine, all of which are stress hormones that activate protective fight or flight responses. These stress hormones can cause hypervigilance, reactivity, fear, worry, and anxiety.

As these SNS-activated emotions become dominant, the prefrontal cortex, the brain's center for thinking and reasoning, becomes increasingly hard to access. The person's capacity for abstract thinking, problem-solving, using good judgment, and self-management is greatly reduced. Under these circumstances, the prefrontal cortex is not able to effectively communicate with the SNS to regulate thoughts, feelings, and behaviors. Excellent and detailed resources for studying this neurobiological activity and trauma can be found in the work of Bessel van der Kolk (2014), Jennifer Sweeton (2019), Rick Hanson (2009, 2013), and Schwartz (2016, 2021).

Self

As we look at these various types of trauma, we see that a fundamental consequence of trauma is damage to self. With the individual's sense of self constantly under fire, they rightfully become self-protective and shut down access to self from others as well as from self. This disconnection from self is one of the most profound effects of trauma. Such disconnection plants the seeds of codependency in some people. By putting us on guard, trauma creates a foundation for external focus. This external focus helps us survive, but it does not give us space and value for developing self-awareness and self-consideration. If we are programmed to constantly watch outside our self for safety, approval, and love, we cannot access and develop our internal connections. There's just no time, space, brain, or heart for doing so.

Clinical Tip Sheet 4: Trauma-Informed Work with Codependency will guide you through trauma assessment and treatment planning with your codependent clients.

Trauma-Informed Work with Codependency

1. **Assessment**

   Assess for traumatic events and symptoms in the intake interview. You can do this in several ways:

   - **Ask about your client's history of abuse, neglect, and losses:** Establish trust and safety as you explore these experiences together. Invite your client's expansion on these events as they are ready and comfortable. As their history unfolds, you can inquire about their symptoms from traumatic events, including both re-experiencing and avoiding responses.

   - **Use J. Eric Gentry's (2021) trauma recovery scale:** https://upstreamcounseling.org/wp-content/uploads/2021/05/BLANK-TRS.pdf. Available in the public domain, this scale is divided into three parts: Part I asks the client if they have had an experience that meets the criteria for PTSD. Part II gathers information about the types of traumatic events, frequency, and dates. Part III assesses the client's symptoms and levels of functioning.

   - **Use the Adverse Childhood Experiences (ACEs) scale (Felitti et al., 1998)** in the public domain and offered here by the National Council of Juvenile and Family Court Judges (2006): https://www.ncjfcj.org/wp-content/uploads/2006/10/Finding-Your-Ace-Score.pdf. Also available in the public domain, you can find more information about the ACEs project at https://www.childhealthdata.org/docs/default-source/cahmi/aces-resource-packet_all-pages_12_06-16112336f3c0266255aab2ff00001023b1.pdf.

2. **Treatment Planning**

   Part III of Gentry's trauma recovery scale can help you and your client determine the level of care they need for the effects of trauma on their life. Once scored, the interpretation of part III provides clear ranges of trauma recovery from full or subclinical to probable traumatic regression. This data can help you and your client decide whether focused, intense trauma work is indicated and how they can get such trauma-informed services from you or through a referral.

3. **Trauma and Codependency**

   As your client recovers from trauma, they will have greater ability to consider self and work on self-understanding *with compassion*. This is when you can, if applicable, help them understand how their loss of self in others may be a natural response to the trauma in their life. Here is a script to help explain these connections.

Psychoeducation Script
Trauma and Codependency

You needed to protect your self from the harm you were experiencing, so you became very externally focused. With your brain's emotional center protecting you, you learned to watch out for people and situations that were dangerous for you—to read rooms, people, and moods—and to keep others happy, to avoid rocking the boat, to do as you were told.

As you developed this strong, protective external focus, you abandoned your self. No blame—of course you did. It was a wise thing to do. There was no time, space, or opportunity for self-awareness, self-knowledge, self-expression, self-confidence, self-trust, or self-compassion.

The good news is that understanding how your trauma history contributes to your codependency can help free you from the effects of trauma. You can learn to safely bring focus to your self and listen and respond to you. When you notice a strong impulse to focus outside your self, this self-understanding can remind you that you now have a choice to abandon self or to attend to self in the new ways you are learning.

Strategy 38

Consider **parts of self** that developed from formative experiences.

The family influences on self-development produce a variety of parts in each of us, parts that may be protective, creative, ambivalent, or counterproductive. Clients often speak in the language of parts intuitively, even if they are not familiar with parts work in therapy:

- "Part of me wants to stay, but part of me wants to go."
- "Part of me hopes they don't see me, and part of me feels ignored."
- "Part of me doesn't want to upset them."
- "Part of me wants it done my way."
- "Part of me feels guilty a lot of the time."

Acknowledging our parts, listening to them, and responding to them are part of self-recovery. There are various ways to work with parts of self, including Schwartz's internal family systems model (IFS; Schwartz & Sweezy, 2020), EMDR, somatic therapies, and gestalt psychology. Such intensive individual therapy can be a part of self-recovery work. Self-recovery supports your client's participation in whatever therapy approach may help them to access self and feel more peaceful and effective.

Handout 12: Parts and Self-Recovery is designed to help you introduce the concept of parts and explore how parts work could support the client's recovery.

Parts and Self-Recovery

Self-recovery is about ultimately developing a relationship-with-self. This involves getting to know the different parts of self. We each have a variety of parts in us, and we often think and speak about them very naturally—for example, "Part of me wants to go out tonight, but another part of me just wants to stay in."

Our parts can serve different roles, and as the parts of self learn to live together in the community of self, an authentic relationship-with-self develops. The following are some examples of the types of parts you may have.

Protective Parts

- **Characters** with specific personalities
  - **Child parts**, some of which include:
    - » Adaptive
    - » Needy
    - » Afraid
    - » Troublemaker
    - » Old voices
    - » Unhappy souls
  - **Adult parts**, some of which include:
    - » Wise self
    - » Ally
    - » Strengths

- **Emotions**, such as:
  - Shame
  - Guilt
  - Fear
  - Loneliness
  - Hope
  - Faith
  - Excitement
  - Regret
  - Delight

- **Thoughts**, such as:
  - *I'm no good.*
  - *Nothing ever works out for me.*
  - *Nobody really cares about me.*
  - *I am not worth caring about.*

- *Bad things will happen if I don't do my part.*
- *I will please them if I do this.*
- *I can add one more thing to my to-do list.*
- *Speaking up is asking for trouble.*

Meeting, Greeting, and Responding to Your Parts

As the parts of self learn to live together in community, an authentic relationship-with-self can develop. In self-recovery work, you are invited to:

- Notice the parts of self as they present themselves, and if possible, name them.

- Establish a connection with the parts by being willing to spend time with them and get to know them.

- Offer curiosity and patience with each part. Quiet your judgment or impatience if you can.

- Listen to what each part wants you to know about them.

- Listen to what the part would like from you here and now.

- Foster a calm back-and-forth conversation with that part guided by a desire for understanding and workability.

- Over time, you will learn how parts can help other parts. For example, if you recognize a part as a child part, your adult parts can attune to the child part and respond with:
  - Listening
  - Reassurance
  - Patience
  - Protection
  - Care
  - Safety
  - Consistency
  - Wisdom
  - Guidance
  - Suggestions
  - Warmth
  - Gratitude

- Your goal is to cultivate a reasonable, responsive, and ongoing relationship with your parts—much as you would with family, friends, neighbors, and even strangers in your community—with your parts learning to work together to foster your developing relationship-with-self.

Strategy 39

Explore **social, cultural, political, and religious influences**.

We now come to the third layer of the circles of influence on self-development: social, cultural, political, and religious influences. The worlds in which we grew up had powerful effects on our beliefs, habits, rituals, traditions, rules, roles, and identity. For example, in terms of codependency, roles assigned based on gender, cultural traditions, or religious beliefs may well have contributed to an imbalance in care of self and others. Patriarchal systems may have limited access to self and discouraged healthy autonomy. Understanding such broader influences promotes our client's compassionate self-understanding by raising their self-awareness and giving them the choice to repeat old patterns or to make changes in self that bring them greater health.

There are a couple of things to keep in mind as you explore this layer of influence with your client. First, the intent is to help them become *aware* of the values, beliefs, norms, teachings, and actions of the worlds in which they were raised. Cultural traditions, religious beliefs, or strong political positions may have been a part of their daily life, woven into their sense of place, purpose, and self.

The second aspect of this work is to be *nonjudgmental* as you and your client recognize what they experienced inside these worlds of school, church, community, clubs, sports, social obligations, government, or work. Judgment can evoke shame, which may already be rooted in these experiences. As an extension of being nonjudgmental, we are not asking our client to change anything they socially, culturally, politically, and religiously believe in and live out, unless they decide it is an obstacle to the growth they seek. Remember, a foundation of self-recovery is helping the client *make their own decisions* about their goals and what changes they are willing and increasingly able to make. Simply understanding self more fully is the intent of this strategy.

The following **Client Worksheet 12: Social, Cultural, Political, and Religious Influences on You** helps you explore and converse with your client about the worlds in which they live.

Social, Cultural, Political, and Religious Influences on You

Study

Look again at **Handout 3: The Circles of Influence on Self-Development**. We have been studying your individual and family influences. Now it is time to take a look at the third layer of influences, the broader worlds in which you grew up—and perhaps still live. These broader influences include your school, church, community organizations, governments, social opportunities, work, and media as well as the traditions, rules, and roles of the culture in which you were raised.

Studying this material helps you become more aware of your broader world experiences and how they may have contributed to your codependency. You will not be asked to change anything you believe in or want to keep in your life. This is simply about becoming self-aware with openness, curiosity, and nonjudgment. Making constructive changes in your life depends on being aware of the working parts that may desire or require adjustments at some point.

Self-Reflection

As you are learning, codependency is about having a dominant focus on others that takes away from a healthy connection with self. The following questions ask about experiences that may contribute to your imbalance in attending to self and others. For each question, please note:

- If that experience was true for you growing up
- If that experience is still true for you today
- Where you had or have that experience: family culture, school, church, community, friends, government, work, media, or some other source

Do any people, places, or events make you feel negated or invisible?

_____

_____

Do any people, places, or events make you feel disrespected?

_____

_____

Do any people, places, or events make you feel restricted from something, unwelcome, or discriminated against?

_____

_____

Do any people, places, or events make you feel like you have to go along with conversations, traditions, roles or tasks that are not true for you?

_____

_____

Do any people, places, or settings make you feel like your time, energy, and needs are not considered or respected?

_____

_____

Do any people, places, or settings feel unsafe for you?

_____

_____

Do any people, places, or settings make you feel you cannot speak your truth?

_____

_____

Do any people, places, or settings make you feel you cannot be who you are?

_____

_____

Looking at these broader influences is powerful. Taking in this fuller picture of you and your life can be overwhelming. It can also be freeing . . . eventually. Perhaps as you reflected on these questions, you noticed an influence that has impacted you for a long time and that you would like to change. Remember, the changes we are working on here are *within you*—how you think, feel, and respond to the worlds in which you live. We are not trying to change these larger systems right here and now; rather, we are trying to help you live in ways that honor and support who you are. We want to help you do that for you.

Notes to Self

_____

_____

_____

Tyler and Self-Understanding

Tyler, 24 years old, was two years into her first serious relationship. She entered counseling, because she was tired of always having to do what her partner wanted to do. Nevertheless, she was very reluctant to speak to her partner directly about her feelings because she was quite afraid she would be abandoned by them. Instead, she kept saying yes when she wanted to say no. Tyler recognized that she was sleeping more than usual and experienced less interest, energy, and pleasure than in the past. She did not want to leave the relationship, but she was not willing to continue to live in her own silence. She felt stuck.

Following her intake interview, Tyler and I took a deeper dive into self-understanding. Her intake interview revealed strong tendencies to please others and avoid conflict, supported by fears of abandonment if she shared her genuine self with her partner. Self-recovery seemed appropriate in order to achieve her goals of finding and using her voice with clarity, confidence, and consideration for her partner and her self.

Tyler enjoyed our exploration of the circles of influence on self-development.

In terms of individual influences, she recognized that her basic nature was quiet and shy. Gentle and soft-spoken, Tyler honored these characteristics as comfortable and appealing to her. She valued her kindness and thoughtfulness.

In term of family influences, Tyler was eager to tell her stories once safety and trust were established with me. Her mother was a functional alcoholic, and her father ignored the problems created by her mother's drinking, which included her mother's yelling, breaking objects, and locking herself in her room. The third child of four, Tyler took on the role of adjuster, always stepping out of the way when conflict occurred. She learned to avoid what was happening and adjust to it. At school, she was an average student who "did not work to her potential," according to teacher reports. Tyler had few friends and was often excluded from lunch tables and social gatherings. She never felt like she fit in anywhere.

As for social, cultural, political, and religious influences, Tyler's family attended church regularly. On Sundays, the family appeared well adjusted and mannered. Other than church, her family went nowhere. They had no friends and did not go on vacations. Tyler's parents saw the world as dangerous and discouraged her from going out in it.

Seeing these influences on her development helped Tyler understand her difficulties in speaking up in her primary relationship and her fears of being left if she was honest with her thoughts and feelings. After all, she had almost no experience doing these things. She had not developed a secure attachment with her parents but rather a combination of insecure avoidant and insecure ambivalent styles, which made her vulnerable to loss of self in others.

Tyler appreciated identifying these influences on self. She agreed that her self-understanding could help her change her habitual relationship patterns of distance, self-protection, and silence as she was ready, willing, and able to do so.

Strategy 40

Address grief that can arise from self-understanding.

As our clients study these influences on self-development, it is not uncommon for grief to set in. In so many ways, these individuals have been naturally protecting themselves from the realities of their formative experiences. In some cases, those experiences may have been helpful and enriching. In other cases, your clients are identifying ways they had to deny self in order to get along, keep the family's status quo, or protect self from harm.

Seeing these realities often involves loss of what they believed, hoped for, or told themselves in order to survive. It may involve loss of relationships, opportunities, or future plans. Grief naturally emerges from this sense of loss. In my work with codependency, I have found that sessions about seeing and accepting the reality of self, others, and situations is heavy work. It is necessary work—the truth will set us free—but first we have to go through the grieving process to get there. As clinicians, we offer a gentle, honest presence with our clients as they grieve. We help them understand they are not giving up hopes and dreams for self; they are seeing and accepting honest data that they can factor into how they consider and respond to self.

I find that Elisabeth Kübler-Ross's (1969) work on grief is helpful, not as stages but as emotional components of grieving. I explain to clients that grief is the name of the umbrella over the emotions of denial, anger, bargaining, depression, and acceptance.

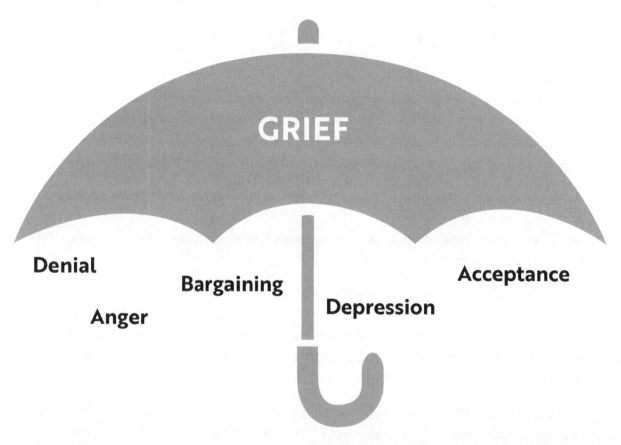

Psychoeducation Script
Grief

Grief involves a variety of emotions. Those emotions can include denial, anger, bargaining, depression, and acceptance. We do not move through these emotions in this order and finally arrive at acceptance. Rather, we move through these components in a random order as we grieve. You may feel one emotion one moment and another the next moment. You may experience acceptance, then find that anger or depression are present again. This is all normal. Of course, we would like to move through grief quickly and in order, but that's not how it happens. Each person's path through grief is different, with its own direction and time frames. We cannot rush grief nor ignore it in the long run.

Most of these five components are self-explanatory, but here are a few details to help you understand their meaning in the context of grief:

Denial can show up even when we know full well something is a fact. Denial creeps in as a thought or feeling like "I just can't believe this is so."

Anger may be toward others, self, or both. It can be a strong emotion that festers, or it may be expressed in hurtful, unproductive ways. Our anger may make sense, or it may involve unmerited blame and regret. Anger often coexists with other feelings, such as love, and makes for confusion and frustration as we try to make sense of conflicting emotions.

Bargaining means looking for something within our control that might have changed the loss we are experiencing. It is often expressed through wishful thinking, such as "If only I had . . ." or "I would do anything if . . ."

Depression can range from manageable to debilitating depending on the extent of our symptoms, which can include sadness, problems with sleep and appetite, reduced energy, interest, and pleasure, and thoughts of our own death.

Acceptance does not mean we like or agree with what is so, but we know it is true and are able to incorporate that truth into the choices we make in our lives. Acceptance can give us strength and freedom.

Let's look together at **Handout 13: Skills for Grieving** to help you with your grief process whenever it may come up.

Skills for Grieving

Grieving is a challenging process. It can be uncomfortable, heavy, and undesirable. We do things to protect our self from grief, even if they may not be best for us. We may let grief eat away at us, causing body and mood problems. We may resort to our addictions to numb the pain of grief. We may act out our grief by making major life decisions too soon, such as moving or ending a relationship, or shutting our self off from people who can safely support us in our grief.

Allowing the grieving process is ultimately helpful. It helps us to move on. It helps us to make informed decisions on our own behalf. It helps us see new choices and possibilities.

When you are ready to allow your grieving process, here are five skills to help you with that. As we look at these skills, let's apply them to the self-understanding you have been gaining:

- **Recognize and name your emotions:** These emotions likely came up for you as you studied the circles of influence on self-development. You have done an amazing job spending time with memories and stories about your relationships with your parents, family, and community. You have taken time to better understand your own basic nature. Have you experienced any of this as loss? Are you aware of emotions such as sadness, anger, frustration? Perhaps you feel relief, clarification, and release. Simply notice, and if possible, name them. Perhaps make a little list of them.

- **Remember that these are not a bunch of unrelated emotions:** The presence of these emotions does not mean that something is very wrong with you. These emotions are all related to grief. Grief can be understood as the "umbrella" over an array of emotions you may be experiencing, including denial, anger, bargaining, depression, and acceptance, as well as others. Your emotions are natural and healing as you let go of something or someone and find your new ways in life. They are all part of change.

- **Allow your emotions:** Recognizing and naming your emotions is great. Now allow your self to be with whatever emotions have arisen. Remember, emotions are parts of you. Acknowledging and owning your emotions can diminish their power. We will work more with emotions in the next chapter on self-awareness.

- **Be with your emotions with safe people, in safe ways:** Your self-understanding will help you put together your pieces of self in new and empowering ways. As you process all of this, it can be helpful to share your emotions with someone who makes you feel safe. Safe means they understand you, care about your growth, and want the best for you. Safe means they respect you and your healing process. When you tell your honest emotions to a safe soul, you can feel connection and understanding, which are healing in themselves.

- **Trust that this grieving process can free you from old patterns and ways of being:** I know this is asking a lot. Trust is a difficult thing to do, especially if our trust has been violated in the past. Here, however, we're referring to developing trust in self. This means learning to listen to and not discount your emotions. It means knowing that what you feel is real and important. It means giving your self permission to experience this process of grief, knowing that it can ultimately soften the pain of your losses.

- **Find meaning in your loss:** David Kessler (2019) identified this important sixth stage in the grieving process. Finding meaning is a personal process and may take time. Meaning can move you beyond acceptance to a vision for self after your loss. Meaning can help you make sense of your grief and transform it into new understandings and strengths that move you forward in your life.

Strategy 41

Address **strengths** identified through self-understanding.

Self-understanding is not only about loss and grief and necessary reconstruction. It can also tap into the strengths upon which we can build if we take time to acknowledge, welcome, and encourage them. As you and your client explore the influences on their self-development, help them notice their strengths revealed along the way. They may be surprised by what they find as they consider their basic nature, family roles, survival, parts, and the broader worlds in which they grew. Here are some examples of strengths revealed through the process of self-understanding:

- **Basic nature:** A client may identify any number of basic traits, including kindness, sensitivity, thoughtfulness, patience, intelligence, cleverness, engagingness, resilience, or tenacity.

- **Family roles:** Strengths can be found within each adaptive family role. Claudia Black (3rd ed., 2020) highlights this well with her roles. For example, someone in the role of the responsible child may be organized, good at decision-making, and self-disciplined. The adjuster may be flexible, remain calm in upsetting situations, and have a strong ability to follow. The acting-out child is honest, experiences their feelings, and may be creative.

- **Survival:** Our clients may have survived unattuned and inconsistent parenting, abuse, neglect, and trauma. Survival invites an important question: "How did you do that? What within you made it possible for you to be here today with me?" A client's strengths gleaned from their survival may include the ability to notice the feelings of others or to read a situation to protect self. It could also be qualities like patience, concern for others, resourcefulness, creativity, determination, and having the belief that they could have a better life in the future. Though the client may already hold these strengths, they may not immediately identify them, and you may need to help them apply this lens of strengths to further heal from their trauma.

- **Parts:** Many of our parts are strengths. Our adult parts, our allies, and our wise parts are important to know and access. They are knowledgeable and eagerly wait for us to remember to consult with them. There are strengths within our child parts as well. They know when we need to take a break or step away from some responsibility. Strengths within our child parts can include humor, playfulness, adventurousness, and spontaneity.

- **Broader worlds:** Your client likely experienced benefits from their broader world influences, even if their circumstances were limiting or negating. Perhaps they developed spiritual strengths through their religious training. Maybe their cultural experiences taught them skills that are useful today. Perhaps their social experiences gave them extra insight and compassion.

As you identify strengths with your clients, remind them that most of their behaviors associated with codependency are valuable traits and qualities that make for a good, engaging life and a content self. The codependent client's challenge is to not allow their strengths to go too far and cause problems for self and others. To see their strengths through an all-or-nothing lens can be problematic. To know, value, and regulate how much they give of their strengths is part of the self-recovery process.

Client Worksheet 13: Identifying Your Strengths can help your client incorporate this important self-knowledge into their accurate sense of self.

Identifying Your Strengths

Study

You have been doing a lot of hard work as you looked at the things that have influenced your self-development. Your strengths can be found within what you are learning. Maybe you have noticed them; maybe there are more inside you that you might be able to discover. Let's take a closer look at your strengths so you can build on them in your self-recovery.

Strengths can be found in your basic nature, in the family roles you took on, in what helped you to survive, in your parts of self, and in benefits from the broader worlds in which you grew up. Look back at your notes on these topics and see what strengths you find. You can start your list with the strengths you are using to do this self-recovery work: diligence, curiosity, openness, hopefulness, and courage. Good work!

Self-Reflection

Name the strengths you've found within your studies on self-understanding.

Strengths in my basic nature include:

_____

_____

Strengths from my family role (or roles) include:

_____

_____

Strengths that helped me survive include:

_____

_____

Some of my parts are strong and wise and are good allies. They include:

_____

_____

Strengths from my experiences with my cultural, social, political, and religious worlds include:

_____

_____

This Week

Stay in touch with your strengths as you move forward with self-recovery. This will help you encourage those strengths and build on them. This week, notice your strengths as they show up. Pay careful attention to how you use your strengths and what it feels like when you lean into them. If your strengths are not naturally showing up in a situation, remember them and call on them.

_____

_____

_____

_____

_____

_____

_____

_____

A word of caution: You can carry your strengths too far. This is when codependency can come into play. Many behaviors associated with codependency are excellent strengths—caregiving, problem-solving, management—but you can overdo these qualities. In so doing, your strengths shift from being assets to causing problems for self and others. As you continue in your healing, you will learn how to maximize your strengths without losing your self in the process.

Notes to Self

_____

_____

_____

_____

Insights and Intentions

Consider the strategies introduced in this chapter:

31. Introduce the **circles of influence on self-development**.

32. Explore **individual influences**.

33. Explore **family influences**.

34. Consider **individuation and differentiation**.

35. Consider **family rules and roles**.

36. Consider **attachment styles**.

37. Consider **trauma history**.

38. Consider **parts of self** that developed from formative experiences.

39. Explore **social, cultural, political, and religious influences**.

40. Address **grief** that can arise from self-understanding.

41. Address **strengths** identified through self-understanding.

What have you learned in this chapter about helping your client develop self-understanding *with compassion*?

_____

_____

Which handouts or worksheets in this chapter seem particularly useful in your work with codependent clients?

_____

_____

Have you had any realizations about your self?

_____

_____

Are there handouts or worksheets from this chapter that you might intentionally bring to your practice or into your own life?

_____

_____

CHAPTER 7

Self-Awareness
Fostered by Calm Presence

Self-awareness, the second element of the four interlocking elements of self-recovery, is needed in each area of self presented in **Handout 9: Four Areas of Self** (p. 53). We will be studying specific strategies for awareness of body, mind, emotions, and spirit in this chapter. But first, we'll start with some foundational information to understand the neurobiology that supports self-awareness.

Self-awareness involves having a calm presence that allows the person to accurately see what is going on and effectively decide what to do for self in that situation. Without calm presence, we are likely reacting rather than responding. When we are anxious, stressed, or fearful, our sympathetic nervous system (SNS) releases adrenaline, cortisol, and norepinephrine, chemicals that activate fight or flight reactions. When our SNS is highly engaged, the prefrontal cortex (our thinking center) has difficulty with rational thinking and decision-making. Additionally, the SNS will not respond to the prefrontal cortex's requests to calm down. These areas of the brain are not able to work together when we are experiencing strong emotions.

Emotional hijacking can be a consequence of the activation of the SNS, one that is especially important to be aware of in work with codependent clients (Schwartz, 2016). As a result of the influences on their self-development, codependent clients can be sensitive and reactive, often anticipating abandonment, fearing conflict, or needing to feel needed. The SNS can be triggered when they experience even a hint of these threatening possibilities.

In addition to fight or flight reactions, there are two less commonly noted SNS reactions—particularly relevant to codependent people—that extend from emotional hijacking. The fawn reaction, which is often related to trauma, involves trying to appease and please the threatening or abusive person (Walker, 2013). Through the person's fawn reaction, they seek safety by merging their wishes and needs with the other person. Another reaction, a variation on the fawn reaction is the *fix* reaction, as discussed by family therapist Terry Real. In a *Relational Life* video, Real (2022) describes this fix reaction not as a thoughtful wanting-to-make-things-better way of being, but as an urgent, compulsive, codependent way of offering *anything* to make the other person feel better.

Whatever reactions your codependent client may have when their SNS is activated—fight, flight, fawn, or fix—it is helpful for them to know the neurobiological reasons for their feelings and their difficulties managing them. This information can reassure them and point them in the direction of calmness and responsiveness. To teach this neurobiology, I created the illustration in **Handout 14: Neurobiology**

and Self. The illustration is a combination of Hanson's (2009, 2013) teachings and my visual way of conveying information. The following psychoeducation script is meant to accompany the handout.

Psychoeducation Script
"The Hot Water Heater and the Lake"

Each of us has an autonomic nervous system that regulates many things in our body and brain. Two parts of that autonomic nervous system are the sympathetic nervous system and the parasympathetic nervous system. Let's look at "The Hot Water Heater and the Lake" in **Handout 14: Neurobiology and Self** to understand what all of this means.

In the center of the illustration is self, represented by the sink with faucets that can draw from hot or cold water. The water pours into the basin of self. We all know that water can scald us and can be uncomfortably cold, and that we can adjust the water faucets so that the temperature works for us. Similarly, we want to adjust our autonomic nervous system so that we have a centered presence from which we can respond, not react, to whatever we are dealing with. A careful look at this illustration will help you understand more about regulating your emotional states.

Let's start with the hot water heater on the left. When we are upset, our sympathetic nervous system (SNS) kicks in and releases stress hormones such as adrenaline, cortisol, and norepinephrine. At a low dose, these hormones are helpful. They produce excitement and energy. At higher doses, they cause stress and worry and result in our fight or flight reactions. The SNS can also cause our emotions to be hijacked, and we may have a fawn or fix reaction to what is threatening us.

Our SNS is protective and designed for our survival. The more alarmed, worried, and distressed we are, the more stress hormones are released to help us protect our self. This natural biological activity heats up the water pouring through the "stress" faucet into the basin of self.

Now look at the lake on the right side of the illustration. It is the water source for the faucet of "well-being." This side of the illustration is about the activity of the parasympathetic nervous system (PNS). This system is naturally in place to calm us, as long as we don't remain in danger or keep thinking and acting in ways to keep the SNS cooking. When we are no longer are in danger, the PNS releases endorphins, natural opioids, nitric oxide, and dopamine to calm and restore us. We can then think and act wisely, use our good judgment, and feel increasingly peaceful.

This image reminds us that we have within us a natural system (the PNS) that can help us adjust the temperature of our stressed, reactive self. There are a number of things you can do to activate your PNS—we will soon learn about these in detail.

Neurobiology and Self*

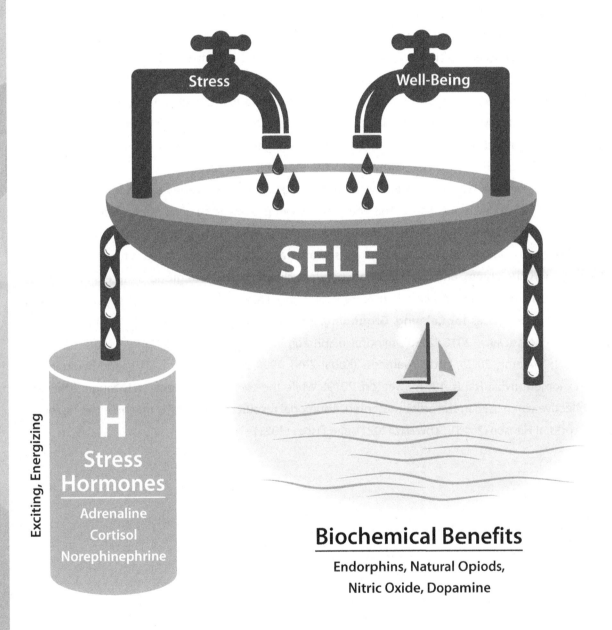

Sympathetic Nervous System (SNS)	Parasympathetic Nervous System (PNS)
Reactive	**Responsive**
Stress, Worry, Anger, Unfulfilled Longings	Pure, Conscious, Peaceful, Radiant, Loving, Wise, Calm

Stress

Well-Being

SELF

Exciting, Energizing

H
Stress Hormones
Adrenaline
Cortisol
Norephinephrine

Biochemical Benefits
Endorphins, Natural Opiods,
Nitric Oxide, Dopamine

---

* Adapted from *Disentangle: When You've Lost Your Self in Someone Else* (2nd ed., p. 251), by N. L. Johnston, 2020, Central Recovery Press.

Strategy 42

Develop **somatic practices** to calm and center.

As we look at self-awareness in each of the four areas of self, let's start with the body. Somatic (body-centered) practices are essential to activating the PNS. When activated, the PNS calms us, quieting the SNS when the prefrontal cortex cannot. As a result, we become more centered and connected once again with self.

Before we go further, a bit more neurobiology will help you understand the somatic practices that follow. The polyvagal theory developed by Stephen Porges (2011) found that the PNS consists of two branches of the vagus nerve: the ventral vagus and the dorsal vagus. Each vagus branch serves a different purpose. In her application of the polyvagal theory to therapy, Deb Dana (2018, 2020) explains these distinctly different branches.

The vagus nerve is divided at the diaphragm. The ventral vagus runs upward from the diaphragm across the lungs and heart, joins with the spine, and travels to the brain. The activation of the ventral vagus restores homeostasis, which includes feeling safe, engaged, and connected.

The dorsal vagus nerve travels downward to the stomach. It is responsible for healthy regulation of the digestive system. When activated by stress or danger, the dorsal vagus can prompt the survival mechanism of a shut down or collapse. This action is another protective survival response from the body, known as the *freeze response*—the person moves out of awareness and away from connection.

For clients to calm, ground, and center their self after activation, they must learn to work with their autonomic nervous system, and providing codependent clients with a core group of accessible somatic practices offers near-immediate ways to increase their internal focus. The following five somatic practices in **Handout 15: Exercises for Calming, Grounding, and Centering** include establishing safety, settling into safe stillness (Dana, 2018, 2020), mindful diaphragmatic breathing (Kabat-Zinn, 1990/2013; Nhất Hạnh, 1991; Sweeton, 2019), body awareness (Kabat-Zinn, 1990/2013; Sweeton, 2019), and being in the present moment (Nhất Hạnh, 1991; Sweeton, 2019). While the exercises are separately taught, they are most effective when used in the order presented. Additional resources for somatic practices can be found in the works of Hanson (2013), Schwartz (2021), and Fisher (2021).

Exercises for Calming, Grounding, and Centering

1) Establishing Safety

Feeling safe is a fundamental need for all of us. Psychologist Abraham Maslow established a hierarchy of human needs. At the top of his pyramid of needs is self-actualization. At the foundation of the pyramid are safety, security, and stability. These foundational needs must be met for us to meet our higher-level needs.

When we feel safe, we are able to be calm and think clearly. New thoughts come to us. We take in the richness of the present moment. With "The Hot Water Heater and the Lake" illustration from **Handout 14: Neurobiology and Self** in mind, we want to activate our parasympathetic nervous system (the lake) so we feel calm and connected with self. Finding safety for our self is a necessary first step in this process of quieting the sympathetic nervous system (the hot water heater).

Practice: You will be making several lists here to raise your awareness of you and safety in your life.

- *Make a list of words or draw images of things that evoke safety for you. Describe why each word or image makes you feel safe.*

- *Make a list of places that feel safe to you. Describe these places. What feels safe about them?*

- *Make a list of people in your life with whom you feel quite safe. What about them makes you feel safe? What do they say or do to convey safety?*

Now, with a safe word, place, or person in mind, notice your body's responses to feeling safe. Describe what you are experiencing, if you can find words for it.

2) Settling into Safe Stillness

Considering the list of behaviors associated with codependency, it is likely you are not used to being still. When we are busy with caregiving, problem-solving, or trying to manage others, being still and quiet is not possible. Tuning into self cannot happen, either. Your external focus probably has your hot water heater turned up higher than is good for you.

Becoming still is an art and a practice that first involves feeling safe. When we can find time and a place of safety to stop and be still, we can naturally begin to tap into that calm lake on a sunny day that is within us. As the hormones of stress and survival are not needed, the body slows down their release. The hormones that produce well-being can then do their part. Our mind can become quieter and our body more relaxed. We have greater access to self.

Practice: Twice each day find five minutes to stop and be still. This can be inside or outside, seated or lying down—wherever you feel safe and will be uninterrupted. I know stillness can be a challenge for people who struggle with codependency. It can feel like a waste of time, or you may worry about what will happen to everyone else while you are being with you. These challenges will subside as you intentionally take time to be still. Let your hands be free of devices; even put them away, if possible. Soon you will learn to bring breath and body practices to your stillness. For now, simply be in silence, allow your body to naturally settle, and invite your thoughts to give you a break.

At the end of your five minutes of stillness, notice how you feel. What was that like? What challenged you in being still? What helped you to be still? Is anything different in you? Do you feel any calmer? Any more connected to you?

3) Mindful Diaphragmatic Breathing

Mindful breathing means paying attention to our in-breath and out-breath. In this practice, we allow our attention to follow our natural breath, not trying to change it or deepen it. In doing this, we are bringing our self into the present moment.

As we follow our breath, it naturally deepens. What begins with the noticing of our breath at our nostrils and mouth can next become noticing our breath at our diaphragm. Eventually we can settle into deep belly breathing. When our diaphragm expands with our in-breath in a safe place, it presses on the ventral vagus nerve, which sends a signal to our brain that is it okay to calm down.

Practice: Find a safe place to become still. Gently shut your eyes or cast your eyes downward.

Settle into your body. If you are seated, place your feet flat on the floor for grounding. If you are seated on the floor, feel your sits bones (those bones on your bottom that you literally sit on) grounding you. If you are lying on the floor, notice the points of your body that are supported by the floor. Notice and try to release any unnecessary holding of your muscles.

Now bring your focus to your breath: Notice the feeling of air coming in through your nostrils. Notice the feeling of air leaving your body, either through your nose or mouth. Notice the natural pauses between your in-breath and your out-breath. Notice the temperature and texture of the air as it comes in and as it goes out. You are not thinking about your breath; you are experiencing your breath. As thoughts run through your mind (which they will), notice them but don't jump on that thought train. Simply redirect your awareness back to the feeling of air coming in and out of your body, here and now.

After a few minutes of following your breath at your nostrils and mouth, shift your awareness of your breath to your diaphragm. Place your hands on your rib cage just above your belly button. Now follow your in-breath as it expands your diaphragm and your out-breath as your diaphragm releases. Settle into the gentle flow of your deep belly breaths at this deeper, safe place within you.

Allow 10–15 minutes for this exercise and do it at least twice per day. You are learning to calm your self and find the entrance to self-awareness.

4) Body Awareness

Settling safely into breath in the present moment opens the door to awareness of sensations in your body. As we have come to know, the body holds much of our tension, unhappiness, and trauma. Learning to listen to the messages from your body can help you identify what you may need to do for you. Is your body tired? Perhaps you need to rest. Is your body agitated? What does it need to calm down? Is your body shut down? What is it asking of you? What parts of you do you notice? Body awareness is an important aspect of cultivating your internal focus.

Practice: Find a safe place to become still. Gently shut your eyes or cast your eyes downward. Settle into following your in-breath and out-breath as you learned in the previous exercise. Do this for five minutes.

Now you are going to do a brief body scan. This means you are going to move through your body in your mind's eye, noticing the sensations in the named part of your body. We will start at your head and move downward to your feet. When you are guided to "notice or feel sensations," this means to pay attention to any tension, tightness, pain, warmth or comfort in that part of your body. Whatever you notice is fine. You are learning how to notice what is going on inside you.

Let's begin.

Notice the top of your head. What sensations do you feel there? What are you aware of? In your mind's eye, breathe in and out through the top of your head.

[What follows is a list of the progression of the body scan through your body. As you move to the next area of the body, use the same guidance offered for the top of the head and continue with *all* areas listed below.]

> *Now shift your awareness to your neck.*
>
> *To your face.*
>
> *To your shoulders.*
>
> *To your arms and down to your hands and fingers.*
>
> *To your spine, traveling through the small of your back to your tail bone.*
>
> *To your heart and lungs.*
>
> *To your stomach.*
>
> *To your hips.*
>
> *Down through your legs to your feet and toes.*

As you near the end of this practice, simply focus on your diaphragmatic breath, imagining it flowing from the top of your head through your body and out through your feet. Stay present with your breath and body in this way for five minutes. Then gently open your eyes and begin to return to the space you are in.

5) Being in the Present Moment

Learning to be safely still, follow your breath, and notice your body sensations are all part of quieting your mind and being in the present moment. This can be quite a challenge for anyone. For codependent people, though, this can be particularly challenging, as you likely spend much time thinking about the past or the future—worrying about what you did or didn't do yesterday and should or shouldn't do going forward. You look outward and forward, not inward here and now. That's okay. Through your self-understanding you are learning why this is true of you, and now with self-awareness, you are learning how you might change this if you wish.

Being in the present moment can be calming and grounding. It gives your "hot water heater" a break and allows the benefits of a cool, beautiful "lake" to pour into you. Then you can think better and work on considering your self as much as you consider others.

Focusing on each of your five senses is another great tool for coming back to the present moment. Our senses of sight, sound, touch, taste, and smell are with us, and they are rich in detail. When you are getting lost in something or someone, you can tune in to one or all your senses to bring you back to you, here and now.

Practice: *Find a safe place to become still. Gently shut your eyes or cast your eyes downward. Settle into following your in-breath and out-breath as you learned earlier, trying especially to notice your diaphragmatic breath. Do this for five minutes.*

Now, open your eyes and pick anything for your sight to focus on. Stay with what you see. Notice the color, the textures, the light, and the details of what you have selected. Spend time taking in that sight. When thoughts show up, nonjudgmentally notice them, then redirect your attention to what you are looking at.

[As you shift to the next sense, continue with a similar pattern through the remaining four senses—choose something to focus on and notice the complex details that each individual sense picks up.]

Now shift your awareness to any sound that may come to your attention.

Now shift your awareness to something you can touch.

Now shift your awareness to something you can taste. Perhaps you have a drink with you. Perhaps you have some residual taste in your mouth.

Now shift your awareness to something you can smell here and now. Perhaps that is some food or drink, hand lotion, soap, or a smell in the room.

Now return to your diaphragmatic breathing for two to three more minutes, letting your experiences with your senses settle in you.

Strategy 43

Teach **cognitive strategies**.

What is your client thinking? Are their thoughts rational and reasonable? Realistic? Unrealistic? Catastrophic? Obsessive? Are they lost in their thoughts? Becoming aware of what is going on in the mind is essential to self-recovery. Cognitive distortions can stop a person from speaking up for self, keep them from believing in their strengths, and be obstacles to change. Becoming aware of the thoughts and beliefs that support their codependent behaviors can help your client adjust their behaviors so those behaviors don't go too far and cause problems for self and others.

In listening carefully to your codependent client, you may reveal their obsessive thinking about any number of things, including how to fix someone else, as well as frequent cognitive distortions similar to those experienced by people in general, including all-or-nothing thinking, overgeneralizing, disqualifying the positive, jumping to conclusions, catastrophizing or minimizing, thinking in terms of "should," and personalizing.

In working with the codependent client, we want to pay attention to their thought distortion and its content. This is how we treat both irrational thinking and codependency. Here are some examples of specific distorted thoughts codependents may express:

- "It's all my fault."

- "I am unlovable."

- "They said I looked good in that color, but they were just being nice."

- "If I don't loan them the money they want, they will never speak to me again."

- "If I say what I think, they will get mad and leave."

- "If I have to leave early, my friends won't invite me to join them again."

As you encounter these errors in thinking in your work with codependent clients, use established techniques from cognitive behavioral therapy (CBT) to help the codependent loosen and modify the messages they are giving themselves (Morrow & Spencer, 2018; Beck, 2021; Burns, 2020). While teaching CBT comprehensively is beyond the scope of this workbook, the next three strategies address specific cognitive distortions of codependent clients and suggest treatment for each of these errors in thinking.

Strategy 44

Become aware of **illusions** about self, the other person, and the situation.

Illusions are inaccurate beliefs, unrealistic expectations, and false hopes, usually about what we think things are or want them to be. Codependent clients can easily become attached to illusions and are hard pressed to let them go. Many years ago, a mentor of mine explained illusions to me as "the glue that hold our crazy-making together." I have quoted her many times because the message within this explanation is so important. Until we recognize our illusions and see and accept the realities of our lives, we stay in the patterns and ways of being that are not serving us.

Seeing and accepting reality is a cognitive and emotional challenge. "Denial" is another word that describes not wanting to see reality. Denial minimizes, discounts, and keeps sending the message that this negative experience will never happen again. Such beliefs keep a person from making changes that may well improve their lives. Breaking through denial and accepting what is will ultimately free us, but before we experience that freedom, we will likely grieve the loss of any number of things brought on by seeing reality, including the loss of hopes, dreams, and perhaps a relationship. Help your client tune in to these losses and work with their grieving process in the ways suggested in **Handout 13: Skills for Grieving** (p. 124).

How will we know when our codependent client is ready to see their reality? First, remember we are working at the pace of our client—where they are in the stages of change, how ready they are to dig deeper, how equipped are they with their essential ingredients of change. Check in with them before you move into talking about the reality of their lives. If you both agree they are ready for this level of honesty with self, **Handout 16: Seeing the Reality of Self, Others, and Your Situation** provides guidance for this work.

Seeing the Reality of Self, Others, and Your Situation

It can be hard to see and accept the realities of who we are and how our life is going. We have a variety of ways we protect our self from those realities, including not thinking about it, denying something happened, or believing something will not happen again. To keep from feeling bad and hopeless, we create illusions. Illusions are beliefs that may or may not be accurate.

Interestingly enough, illusions also keep us from growing. Our beliefs, whether they are accurate or not, keep us saying and doing the same old things. We remain stuck in our patterns of how we relate to other people and how we treat our self. Though it can be hard at first, learning to see and accept what is can free you.

Facing your illusions can help you have more accurate thoughts and expectations so you don't keep falling into the same holes.

Here are some ways to help you look at your beliefs and determine whether they are illusions or not.

1. **Identify your beliefs:** Here are some beliefs codependent clients tell themselves:

    *   **Beliefs about Others and Our Relationship with Them**
        1. "They can't do this without me."
        2. "They need me to help in this way."
        3. "They will leave me if I don't do this."
        4. "They will fail if I don't help."
        5. "If I say it enough times, they will get it."

    *   **Beliefs about Self**
        1. "I am so caring and helpful."
        2. "I only want what's best for them."
        3. "I am not angry."
        4. "I don't expect anything in return."
        5. "I can't live without them."

    Do you identify with any of these beliefs? Do other beliefs of your own come to mind?

2. **Study the accuracy of your beliefs:** Pay honest attention to you, the other person, and your situation:

    *   Consider whether there is any objective data to support your beliefs.

    *   See you and the other person as you are here and now.

    *   Notice words and actions in the present moment.

    *   Stop making excuses for, defending, or rationalizing what is.

    *   Notice your feelings, thoughts, and behaviors in the present moment.

- Allow your self to take all of this in, not confronting the other person but rather absorbing the realities you may find.

- Take your realizations to your journal, your therapist, or your trusted guide to process your more accurate and honest thoughts and feelings.

3. **Make more accurate and honest statements to self:** Once you have studied the accuracy of your beliefs, create a new, realistic statement to self. Here are some examples:

- **Realities about Others and Our Relationships with Them**
    1. "They can do this without me."
    2. "I know they can do this on their own, but it probably won't be the way I would do it."
    3. "I must do this for me, even if they leave me."
    4. "My help really isn't keeping them from failing in the long run."
    5. "My repeating myself will not make things better."

- **Realities about Self**
    1. "I am caring and helpful, and I am trying to have things my way."
    2. "I really don't know what is best for them."
    3. "I am angry."
    4. "I will be disappointed if they aren't grateful."
    5. "I can live without them."

Look back at one of the beliefs you named earlier in this exercise. Study the accuracy of that statement, then create an honest, accurate statement you can use to help you make the changes you want for you.

Strategy 45

Learn to **separate** problems and issues of others from those of self.

Another cognitive distortion codependent clients may experience is not knowing where they end and the other person begins. There can be such physical and emotional enmeshment between the codependent and others in their life that the mental distinction of what is mine and what is yours is not present. The codependent's beliefs support this enmeshment:

- "I know what is best for them."
- "I did it even though they did not ask me to."
- "The argument was completely my fault."
- "I am the one with the problem."
- "If I weren't so _____, they would be happier with me."
- "I can fix this person."
- "If I fix them, I will be fine."

When your client is ready, they can begin to mentally separate the pieces of self from their enmeshed relationship. This begins with the cognitive task I call the "line down the page exercise"—literally drawing a line in the middle of a piece of paper with *My Problems/Issues* on one side of the line and *Their Problems/Issues* on the other side of the line. **Client Worksheet 14: Separating Me from You** walks you and your client through this exercise.

A variation of this worksheet exercise can be done seated in your office with your client. When I realize this visual of "the line down the page" may help a client, I introduce it by gesturing a vertical line from top to bottom in space. Then I use the following script to guide them through the exercise:

Psychoeducation Script
"The Line Down the Page"

You are on one side of this line. On the other side of the line is the person you are concerned about or involved with. The line is not a wall. It is simply where you end and where the other person begins. You can take anything you want to the line: a statement, a gift, a request, an idea. Then, you leave what you have offered and step back, giving them space to listen and consider what they want to do with what you have laid out there.

Be careful not to try to push you and your offering further onto their side by insisting, elaborating, or volunteering to do what they should do. Stay steady with you. Back further from the line if you find your self repeating or explaining more. Reassure your self that you are fine with what you have delivered and will be okay if the other person does not pick it up. It is theirs to do with as they choose.

Return your focus to your feelings, needs, and desires for you and your day.

This gets easier the more you do it.

Separating Me from You

Study

This worksheet can help you sort out *you* from a person with whom you may be entangled. When you have lost your self in someone else, it can be hard to separate you from them. Seeing what is yours and what is not can help you change your habitual patterns and improve your mental health.

Think of someone with whom you are entangled. Choose a specific problem or issue that entangles you (e.g., getting housework, homework, or projects completed or scheduling medical appointments).

With this entanglement in mind, fill in the *My Problems/Issues* column with your responsibilities, desires, feelings, and actions. When you stumble into items for the other person—their responsibilities, desires, feelings, and actions—jot them down in the *Their Problems/Issues* column.

After you've completed the two-column chart, use this information to address the questions in the next section of this worksheet.

My Problems/Issues	Their Problems/Issues

Self-Reflection

Working with the problem or issue you identified, what are the items in your own column you would like to focus on? What are things in your column you can do something about? What can you take action on now?

_____

_____

_____

_____

What draws you to the other person's column? What thoughts have you looking over the line at them or stepping further into their column?

_____

_____

_____

_____

Are you interested in spending more time and energy on your side of the line?

_____

_____

_____

_____

This worksheet is to help you see how you may be taking on more than is yours. It shows you where you are putting your thoughts and energy and where you could be offering more to your self.

Notes to Self

_____

_____

_____

_____

Strategy 46

Teach **healthy detaching**.

This cognitive distortion arises from being in such a strong emotional state that the person is not able to think clearly—or hardly at all. We studied this neurobiological reality earlier in this chapter using **Handout 14: Neurobiology and Self** (p. 133). When our SNS is activated by stress, threat, or danger, the flood of adrenaline, cortisol, and norepinephrine make it difficult to use our prefrontal cortex for thinking and decision-making. Quieting our "hot water heater" is essential to being able to think more clearly and effectively. Without doing so, we can have multiple errors in our thinking and judgment.

Codependent individuals are inclined to be reactive, not responsive. Our wiring has us protectively defending, deflecting, projecting, or collapsing. Healthy detaching is about finding emotional and cognitive balance for self. It is not necessarily about leaving or ending a relationship. Instead, it is about becoming clear and centered, calm, and able to think. As we do this, we can see the reality of self, the other person, and the situation, and we can make better decisions about what to do in the moment or for our future. We can then speak and act with that clarity grounding and centering us.

Handout 17: Quieting Your Emotions So You Can Think Better offers four skills you can teach your client to quiet their fight/flight/freeze/fawn/fix reactions and increase their ability to think effectively on their own behalf.

Quieting Your Emotions So You Can Think Better

1) Get Centered

When we feel upset, hurt, or threatened, our body responds by setting off our survival alarms. Those alarms prompt us to fight or flee; fawn or fix; or freeze, but when they are blaring their warnings, it is almost impossible to think. Clear thinking promotes effective care of self. So let's turn down those neurobiological alarms. You can do this by using the somatic exercises on safety, stillness, breath, body, and present moment from **Handout 15: Exercises for Calming, Grounding, and Centering**.

When we have grown up externally focused, we tend to be unaware or unacquainted with our centered self, who readily offers wisdom, comfort, and clarity. But we have the power to center our self—"getting centered" means bringing focus to your self and becoming stable and secure through that internal connection. You check in with all four areas of self.

> *Practice:* When you find your self dominantly other-centered and your alarms are going off, notice the alarms. Then pause and reconnect with you. Use somatic practices to create a safe, calm presence for you. Then tune in to you: what are you feeling, needing, and wanting in this situation? Find your center by focusing on both what is happening outside of you and within you.

2) Observe

With our centeredness, we are able to observe the other person and our self in the present interaction. We take in what and how the other person is saying or doing. We pay attention to what we are thinking and feeling. We quiet judgment and bring in patience and objectivity. We check in with our motivations in the situation. We become honestly aware of what we are trying to accomplish in our interactions with this person. We are trying to gain an accurate and full understanding of what is happening.

> *Practice:* Once you have centered your self in a conflictual interaction, use your emotional and cognitive balance to observe rather than jumping right in. To set this up, say to your self: "Just listen. Stay calm. Observe. Think. Take your time. Release pressure. Breathe. Stay with self."
>
> With this observational stance established, you can then take in what the other person is saying and doing, as though the person were on a stage or television. You can also take in what you are thinking, feeling, and how your body is reacting. Just observe. Your centeredness and this more objective data can help you discern what you want to say or do.

3) Respond, Don't React

The suggestions to get centered and observe prepare us to *respond* instead of react. When we are frightened, threatened, or feeling under attack, it is natural to react in defensive ways. If the situation is indeed dangerous, it is essential that we follow our survival instincts. However, if you wish to respond to your situation with a clear head and grounded intent, begin by getting centered and observing.

As we safely calm, center, and observe, we will be able to formulate thoughts and sentences and deliver them in assertive tones to the other person. Meeting attack with attack won't help this conversation a bit. Defensiveness breeds defensiveness. When we respond rather than react, we are representing our self in solid and effective ways. We have the ground under our feet and access to our thoughts, feelings, and actions.

Practice: Think of an interaction you had recently that was strongly emotional for you. Pick an example in which you reacted more than responded. We all do this. Now, pause, breathe, and consider how you might have honestly responded to the other person. What were you feeling? What thoughts were in your head? Be careful not to say to your self, "Oh, I feel so ashamed. I should have known to _____." That is external thinking. You are invited here in the safe calm of this moment to identify what was true for you and what you might have said or done to represent you.

4) Use Self-Talk

Anchoring our self through self-talk is an effective way to stay centered. Self-talk is an established cognitive behavioral technique. It can take the form of reminders, affirmations, reassurances, or simply restatements to self. With codependency, we can be so pulled off our center as we interact with someone else that we become confused, frustrated, and lost. Self-talk can help us stay connected to the centeredness we have found through the first three skills in this handout.

Examples of anchoring self-talk statements include:

- "I'm okay."

- "It is okay to say this."

- "I haven't done anything wrong."

- "This is not my issue."

- "I am not the problem. I don't want to become the problem."

Self-talk can also take the form of an internal dialogue that may be as active as the external dialogue you are having. While you are talking with someone else, you can simultaneously have your own conversation with your self, helping you stay clear and representing your self fairly.

Practice: Let's plan in advance of conflict. What are some self-talk statements that are true for you in general? For example, "I mean no harm," "It is okay for me to say what I think," or "It is important for me to say what I need." Remember, these are statements from you to you. These are not statements to say to the other person in the middle of your interaction with them. Wake up your mind to such self-supportive messages. Practice them throughout your day as you converse with you and interact with others.

Strategy 47

Increase **emotional awareness and expression**.

We are always experiencing emotions, whether we are aware of them or not. Often, we are not aware in a conscious, responsible way. Even if we have some awareness of our feelings, we discount, minimize, or rationalize them. Some emotions may feel overwhelming, and we fear we will be stuck in that emotion if we acknowledge and allow it.

In working with clients on self-awareness of emotions, the third area of self, I have heard many describe these concerns. When this happens, I honor the client's worries, recognizing how powerful emotions can be, and inform them that they have many options for bringing emotions into awareness and handling them in informed ways. **Handout 18: Healthy Emotional Expression** illustrates the flow of emotional awareness and the choices available to your client for regulation and expression of their emotions as they are ready.

Psychoeducation Script
Emotional Awareness and Expression

Let's look at **Handout 18: Healthy Emotional Expression**. Think of this chart as a menu of options for managing your emotions. As you see, the top bar says "Feelings – Emotional Awareness – Choices."

Feelings

Let's start with feelings. We all have feelings most of the time. Sometimes we are aware of them. Often, though, they are just outside our awareness. Sometimes we feel them in our body but push them away or say, "I shouldn't feel that way." Sometimes we have no idea what to do with them. They may be scary, bothersome, or distracting. They may be positive or hopeful. Knowing that you have feelings most of the time is important in itself. Feelings are waiting there for you to notice them so you can understand and respond to your emotions.

[**Note to Clinician:** Pause and discuss with your client this section about feelings. Then invite them to apply in session what you are teaching them as you travel through this script together.]

Emotional Awareness

Now let's talk about bringing your feelings into your emotional awareness.

- **Become aware:** When you feel ready, open your self to how your body is feeling, what your thoughts are telling you, and what emotions are arising here and now. Settle into your diaphragmatic breath as you join these internal experiences. Do your body sensations help you understand what emotions you are experiencing? Do your thoughts match your emotions? Stay with your internal experiences to better discern your honest emotions at this time.

- **Recognize:** Do you recognize the emotions that are within you? Is the emotion familiar? Does it make sense to you in light of what is going on right now? Or is it an old feeling that keeps showing up? Perhaps you recognize a general emotional state such as sad, angry, or happy.

- **Identify:** Now see if you can specifically name the emotions you are aware of. For example, if you recognize the emotion as sad, can you go further to see if that means disappointed or hopeless? If your emotion is happy, do you feel calm or encouraged? I will stay with you as you dig deeper to call your emotions by name as best you can. Acknowledging your emotions is a healthy foundation for taking care of them.

  [**Note to Clinician:** Take as much time as your client needs to name their emotions. This is a step-by-step process of gaining emotional awareness. When your client is ready to study the choices they have for emotional expression, continue with this script.]

Choices

Here are five different ways you can manage and express your emotions. No one way is better than another. As you become familiar with these strategies to handle your emotions, you will know which is the better choice for you in a particular situation at that time.

- **Chaperone or be with:** Thích Nhất Hạnh (1991), a Buddhist monk who brought mindfulness practices into everyday life, teaches us to recognize our feeling and then breathe mindfully as a way of calming our self and being with our feeling. He suggests we attend to our feeling in the way we would care for a baby. We tenderly hold our feeling as a parent would hold their child. As we become calm, so does our feeling. We can then let go of the feeling. The final step is to look deep into the causes and nature of the feeling. This opens the door to transforming the feeling.

  [**Note to Clinician:** Pause and invite discussion and practice of this strategy.]

- **Cues and signals:** Sometimes our emotions are sending us an important self-care message that we would do well to hear. Emotions let us know how we feel about the way we are being treated. They alert us to the types of care we may need to give to our body or to our spirit. They provide information to help us make decisions that are in our best interest. Yes, sometimes our feelings come from misperceiving something or someone, but even in such cases, it's healthy to explore what those feelings may be signally for you. Emotions can also signal the need for us to *HALT*: Am I <u>H</u>ungry? <u>A</u>ngry? <u>L</u>onely? <u>T</u>ired? Whether you have one or all of these feelings, this valuable acroynm directly tells you to stop, regroup, and restore self.

  [**Note to Clinician**: Pause and invite discussion and application of this strategy.]

- **Contain:** Sometimes emotions are so strong that we don't yet know what to do with them. For example, you may open up about your emotions here in a session, but we may not be able to transform them in that same session. Neither of us wants you to carry them around with you like an open wound until we meet again. "Containing" those emotions means finding a way, a place, or a process by which you can set the emotions down until you wish to pick them up again. Some examples of containment include leaving your emotions on the pages of your journal, imagining placing them on a shelf or in a drawer, or leaving them in this office until you return and wish to take them out again. Knowing that you can manage your emotions in this way helps you safely access them, yet not carry them around with you so that they influence your days and relationships.

[**Note to Clinician:** Pause and invite discussion. See if your client can identify a safe way for them to contain their emotions. How do they feel about this idea?]

- **Communicate:** Once you have identified an emotion and have a calm presence with it, your may find that you want to communicate your emotion to someone else. Healthy communication is paramount in our relationships. If you choose to communicate your emotion, first rehearse what you want to say with someone who is safe, someone who understands the work you are doing and supports you. (That could be me.) This rehearsal will help you clarify what you want to say and how to say it. There are specific skills to help you express your self that we will be studying in self-competence, the next element in self-recovery. For now, know that communicating your emotion can be a healthy choice.

[**Note to Clinician:** Pause and invite discussion. Ask your client if they have an emotion they would like to try to communicate to you here and now.]

- **Change neural structure:** When we consider our reluctance to acknowledge emotions, we are often referring to feelings that disturb us or cause us pain. But we can also have bright, kind, encouraging feelings that we may not want to attend to, either. We dismiss compliments. We don't accept someone's offer of help. We receive good feedback but tell our self it was not good enough or the person doesn't really mean what they are saying. Codependent individuals can have a particularly hard time letting these good feelings seep in. Our sense of self does not have space for this positivity. As you gain self-recovery, however, this can change. Rick Hanson (2009, 2013, n.d.) is a psychologist who teaches that by allowing the good to seep in, we can become more aware of and receptive to positive experiences in our life. By absorbing your good feelings and experiences, you can actually change your brain structure in a direction that promotes emotional balance rather than fight/flight/fawn/fix/ freeze responses. Imagine that!

[**Note to Clincian:** Pause and discuss. Then offer your client the opportunity to identify and absorb a positive feeling. Take 10 to 30 seconds (or more) to let that good seep in (Hanson, n.d.).]

Healthy Emotional Expression*

Pathways to Emotional Health

FEELINGS	EMOTIONAL AWARENESS	CHOICES

Chaperone/Be With
- Hold feeling in gentle awareness
- Support it with mindful presence

Cues/Signals
- Self-care
- HALT (hungry, angry, lonely, tired)

Become Aware

Feeling **Recognize** ### Contain

Identify ### Communicate
- To others you feel safe around
- To the person involved, assertively

Change Neural Structure
- Negativity bias to positivity
- Let the good seep in

---

* Adapted from *Disentangle: When You've Lost Your Self in Someone Else* (2nd ed., p. 252), by N. L. Johnston, 2020, Central Recovery Press.

Strategy 48

Increase awareness of **spiritual sources**.

My inclusion of spirituality as the fourth and final area of self began with my recovery in a twelve-step program. Twelve-step programs are not religious, but they do invite a belief in a power greater than self. Through my codependency recovery, I became aware of my needs to manage and control others. Robin Norwood (1985/2008) brought that to my attention in her book *Women Who Love Too Much*, in which she includes the cessation of managing and controlling others as one step to recovery from loving too much (losing self in others). As I worked with my controllingness, the twelve-step program I attended for family and friends of alcoholics gave me important tools for letting go of things over which I have no control; one of those tools is releasing what I can't control to something beyond me. (We will work on this letting-go process in the chapter on self-attunement.)

Spirituality has continued to grow in importance to the self-recovery process. In the calm presence that can come from grounding and centering practices, there is space for connection with not only thoughts and feelings but also with something beyond self. Such spiritual experiences cannot necessarily be named or taught, but we can introduce the idea and value of spirituality and see the ways our clients may be open to it.

For people with religious beliefs, their greater power will most likely be the god of their faith. Helping them find ways to join their religious beliefs with their self-recovery can be quite powerful. Their beliefs may well be a source of strength and comfort for them that create the safety needed to calm and access self. Religious beliefs may also offer a trusted outlet beyond the individual for letting go of things they cannot control. Working with your client to see how their religious resources can safely support their self-recovery can strengthen self-integration.

For people with no defined religious beliefs, spirituality may be an experience unique to them. They may find something beyond self in nature, friends, silence, the universe, the present moment, or simply a feeling or an experience that defies easy description.

Gut feelings and intuition can fall within this spiritual category. We want to help our client to not dismiss these messages with their rational brain or strong emotions. Spending time with these less tangible parts is important for attending to their more complete self. Their gut feelings and intuition are likely relaying messages to help with discerning, deciding, and changing.

There will also be clients who are not comfortable with this area of spirituality. Their life experiences may have them staying away from anything that seems like religion, or they may simply not grasp or appreciate this idea of spirit itself. In these cases, introduce the material as I am introducing to you here, then join your client to decide how they want to use what is being offered. They will find their way. In a sense, this is a demonstration of spirituality in action: we offer, they listen, and we let go with trust and space for their own discerning and growth.

Self-recovery recognizes spirituality within us. It is a wise part of us we can know, cultivate, and come to trust. That spiritual part invites our questions with patience and presence. It can provide loving and helpful internal guidance to discern what is true for us and what will enrich and stabilize our life. Our interactive engagement with our spiritual source can offer:

- A calming presence

- A safe relationship

- Space to connect with self

- Space to connect with something beyond self

- Something constant and reliable

- Something to call upon

- Something to let go to

Client Worksheet 15: Spirituality and You introduces spirituality to your client and gives them an opportunity to explore their relationship with it.

Spirituality and You

Study

Spirituality means different things to different people. In this moment, we are speaking about spirituality as "something beyond self." A person's spirituality is an individual choice. Some people have religious beliefs as their spiritual sources. Others may find their spirituality in nature, friendships, silence, the universe, a song, a time of day—any number of things. Gut feelings and intuition can serve as spiritual sources for some. And some people do not subscribe to the belief in something beyond self.

Spirituality can offer us a calming presence; a safe relationship; something constant, reliable, and wise; something to call upon; and something to let go to. It can offer us space to connect with self and with something beyond self.

In this worksheet, you are invited to explore your self and spirituality. There is no intent other than to help you increase your self-awareness about this fourth area of self.

Self-Reflection

Take a moment to consider spirituality in your present life. Is spirituality present? If yes, what form does it take? If not, how do you feel about this topic of spirituality?

_____

_____

How do you make contact with your spirituality? How often and under what circumstances?

_____

_____

Is spirituality important to you? Does it make a difference in your life?

_____

_____

Would you like to make any changes in your connection with your spiritual self? Would you like to foster your relationship with your spiritual sources?

_____

_____

How might this help you?

_____

_____

What might you do to develop your spiritual self?

_____

_____

How are you feeling about this inclusion of spirituality in your self-recovery?

_____

_____

Notes to Self

_____

_____

_____

_____

Tyler and Self-Awareness

Gaining self-awareness was a new venture for Tyler. Having been the adjuster in her family system while growing up, Tyler was good at stepping out of the way of conflict, rejection, and inconsistency. In order to live this role, she had to ignore her own thoughts, feelings, and wishes.

Tyler enjoyed the calm space of our counseling work. She often remarked on how odd it felt to be listened to and acknowledged. As she settled into this safety, we began self-awareness with the illustration of the four areas of self. Tyler said she had never teased out these areas before. She had always felt like "one big mess." Her best choice, she said, had been to "ignore it all."

Using a number of the handouts and worksheets in this chapter, Tyler made solid progress in self-awareness:

- **Body:** *Though she was quiet, Tyler recognized that she was usually tense and tight. She took to the somatic practices, especially the* **diaphragmatic breath** *and* **body scan**. *She was amazed at how calm she became and how much clearer her thoughts were when she used these practices.*

- **Mind:** *Tyler realized that some of her inability to speak up to her partner came from having a blank mind or not knowing what she wanted to say. She especially liked the skills for* **detaching,** *where she learned to* **observe** *her partner as they communicated,* **calm** *her self so she didn't shut down, and use* **self-talk** *to know what she honestly wanted to say in response.*

- **Emotions:** *Tyler had little connection with her emotions. Believing that her quiet, adjusting ways protected her from her feelings, she was surprised to find strong emotions within. Counseling offered her a safe place to identify emotions such as anger and loneliness. Tyler learned to* **be with or chaperone** *her feelings and enjoyed discovering what* **cues** *her emotions gave her about her needs and wants.*

- **Spirit:** *Tyler did not enjoy attending church with her family as a child and had doubts about religion and its purpose in her life. She was attracted to the idea that spirituality does not necessarily involve religious beliefs. She had always enjoyed walks on her own, especially in nature. She was comforted by them and felt connected with a world broader than just her room. She increased the frequency of her nature walks and started to pay attention to her gut feelings and intuition, which she previously had no awareness of.*

Insights and Intentions

Consider the strategies introduced in this chapter:

42. Develop **somatic practices** to calm and center.

43. Teach **cognitive strategies**.

44. Become aware of **illusions** about self, the other person, and the situation.

45. Learn to **separate** problems and issues of others from those of self.

46. Teach **healthy detaching**.

47. Increase **emotional awareness and expression**.

48. Increase awareness of **spiritual sources**.

What have you learned in this chapter about helping your client develop self-awareness *fostered by calm presence*?

_____

_____

Which handouts, worksheets, or scripts in this chapter seem particularly useful in your work with codependent clients?

_____

_____

Have you had any realizations about your own self-awareness in any or all four areas of self?

_____

_____

Are there handouts, worksheets, or scripts from this chapter that you might intentionally bring to your practice or into your own life?

_____

_____

CHAPTER 8

Self-Competence
with Increasing Confidence

Welcome to the third element of self-recovery: self-competence *with increasing confidence*. This is where we help our codependent clients develop skills needed for the shift from their strong external focus to their attentive, responsive internal focus. These skills support and extend the work they have already been doing with self-understanding and self-awareness. We can understand our self better and know how to safely calm our self, but the nuts and bolts of managing guilt and setting boundaries, for example, often need to be taught. Once learned, we become more competent and confident in our abilities to balance self and other and take good care of self.

We have already studied skills involved in grief processing, strength identification, and numerous skills to increase self-awareness. In this chapter, we will study healing shame, managing guilt, assertiveness, and boundary setting. I have intentionally put these skills in this order. If I teach boundary setting first, my codependent clients' needs for guilt management and assertiveness show up. If I introduce any of these skill sets before we address healing shame, clients bring their feelings of unworthiness and undeservedness to any assertions for self.

Strategy 49

Practice **five foundational skills**.

Before we study these skill sets for shame, guilt, assertiveness, and boundaries, we must get familiar with five skills that are foundational to each of these skill sets:

1. Pausing and stopping

2. Mindful breathing

3. Quieting thoughts

4. Releasing body tension

5. Being in the present moment

These are the somatic practices taught in self-awareness, and they create a solid self-foundation that will support your client's use of the new skill sets as they learn the strategies that follow. These foundational skills help your client access self so they can then remember and use the new skills they are acquiring.

On the next page is **Handout 19: Five Foundational Skills**. These five foundational skills set the stage for your client's recovery work every time they practice them. Share it with them in session and practice each of the skills regularly in your work together.

Five Foundational Skills

These five skills help you establish your connection with self, which then makes it possible for you to remember and use the skill sets you will be learning for self-recovery. Practice these foundational skills often so they are there for you when you really need them.

1) Pausing and Stopping

Pause. Stop. This is an intentional act that interrupts whatever you may be thinking or doing and gives you space within to connect with you. Your intentional pause opens the door to each of the other four foundational skills,

2) Mindful Breathing

Notice the experience of air coming in and out of your body either at your nostrils or your diaphragm. Follow your breath for four or five cycles, settling into the calm this can offer.

3) Quieting Thoughts

As you follow your breath, you will notice thoughts running through your head. This is normal. Notice those thoughts, but don't join them. Simply redirect your focus back to your inhalations and exhalations. You are not only calming down, but you are also creating space within you to help you listen to and respond to self.

4) Releasing Body Tension

As you settle into your breath and quiet your thoughts, scan your body for tightness or unnecessary holding. Breathe in and out of these areas, releasing the tension you may find there. You are resetting your self so you can think and act in new ways.

5) Being in the Present Moment

Each of these foundational skills are about coming out of an interaction or out of your head and into the present moment. An additional way to be present is to tune in to your senses. Really notice how food tastes, see the sky, or smell your coffee. This present moment awareness restores your connection with self and gives you the opportunity to choose how you want to handle a situation or what is best for you.

Strategy 50

Learn to **transform shame**.

Some clients are aware of their shame, while others are not. Some knowingly carry shame as a burden, unaware they can heal and release it, allowing for fresh growth for self. Some are stuck in self-sabotaging patterns, unaware that shame is feeding the destructive behaviors they would like to change. Either way, shame is alleviated by being brought into the light of day in a safe place with a trusted person.

Codependency is often accompanied by shame and guilt. The difference between these feelings, simply put, is that guilt is the feeling of having done something wrong, while shame is feeling that something is wrong with you, that you are broken, unworthy, and unfixable.

To begin understanding the relationship between shame and codependency, let's look at Brené Brown's "shame shields" (2007, 2018). Building from the work of relational-cultural theorist Linda Hartling, Brown identifies three responses to shame that attempt to cope with the pain of feeling broken and unworthy. (Hartling refers to these responses as "strategies of disconnection"; you will also recognize them as responses to activation of the sympathetic nervous system.)

- We move *against* shame by fighting back, by using shame to fight shame (i.e., fight)

- We move *away from* shame by withdrawing, hiding, being silent (i.e., flight)

- We move *toward* shame by trying to appease, people-pleasing (i.e., fawn)

Any of us can use any of these shame shields at various times, depending on the person and situation. Of particular note, though, is the third shield of *moving toward* shame by appeasing and pleasing. While all codependents do not present in this fawning way, for many, this is their habitual interpersonal pattern—to appease and please others, not self. This supports our clinical community's growing understanding that codependency is often a self-protective response to shame and trauma. In other words, it is often shame that causes the codependent to carry their codependent behaviors too far, shame that makes it uncomfortable to increase internal focus, shame that makes it difficult for the codependent client to believe they are worthy of a relationship-with-self.

Shame in the codependent client may originate in any and all of the circles of influence on self-development. The individual's shame may have been instilled through childhood experiences or messages that made them feel broken or unworthy. They may have received conditional love from their family or been neglected or abused. They may have been told they deserved the harsh treatment they were receiving. They may have learned they are not valuable and loveable. Additionally, the social, cultural, political, and religious worlds in which they lived may have encouraged self-abandonment and may have been outright traumatic. Shame festers from these sources, growing into a heavy weight that is carried in the soul and shows up daily in how the codependent person relates to others and to self.

Handout 20: Shame and Codependency invites your client to consider their inner experience of shame and the ways it expresses itself in their lives.

Shame and Codependency

Shame is feeling like you are broken, that something is very wrong with you and cannot be fixed. Shame feels like you are unworthy or not enough. Shame is also very good at hiding itself—you may or may not be aware of your shame. Becoming aware of your shame and bringing it out of hiding with safe people can open the doors to deep healing.

We will go slowly as you consider meeting your shame. A good place to start is becoming aware of how it shows up in your daily life, how it may be running the codependency show without your awareness. Here are some examples for us to study and discuss:

- Because you believe you are **broken**:
  - You don't ask for much or expect much from others.
  - You prefer to keep your focus on others rather than be with what you experience as your brokenness.
  - You believe your brokenness cannot be fixed, so you put your energy into fixing others: "I am okay if you are okay."
  - You discard self like a broken item: thrown away, put in a drawer, garage, or attic, never to be revisited again.

- Because you feel like you are **not enough**:
  - You do too much for others to prove your value, to have a purpose, to have a place.
  - You fill your schedules to fill your self.
  - You don't say no, hoping your yes will make you more valuable and complete.
  - You engage in addictive behaviors such as shopping, spending, engaging in relationships, using substances, and eating food, to bring pleasure and completeness to your self.

- Because you feel **unworthy**:
  - You feel less than others: *Doesn't matter what I think.*
  - You don't ask for help: *Not worth it.*
  - You don't ask to be treated fairly: *Don't deserve it.*
  - You don't expect much: *Why should I?*
  - You don't deserve much: *Of course not.*
  - You don't prioritize self: *Too busy. Why bother?*

Understanding the relationship between shame and codependency is an important start to lessening and releasing these powerful undercurrents in your life.

If your client finds shame within themselves, the following psychoeducation script on transforming shame can assist with education, exploration, conversation, insight, and release.

Psychoeducation Script
Transforming Shame

Brené Brown's work (2007, 2018) has done much to advance our understanding of shame and what can transform it. A major emphasis in her research is the individual's move from shame to empathy, from a place of fear and disconnection to a place of compassion and connection. Shame tends to hide out and keep itself secret. But when it is *met with empathy and understanding, it loses its destructive power.*

Brown (2007) established the shame resilience theory, which identifies four elements in transforming shame: (1) recognize and understand your shame triggers, (2) develop critical awareness about your shame and its sources, (3) become willing to reach out to safe others, and (4) speak to safe others about your shame.

When teaching shame resilience, I make a few adjustments to Brown's original theory. First, I add the word *safe* to the elements regarding reaching out and speaking to others to reinforce this important therapeutic piece involved in self-recovery: be willing to reach out to *safe* others and speak to *safe* others about your shame. It's important to share this vulnerable part of our self with people whom we consider trustworthy. I also add a fifth and final element to Brown's list: release your shame. Releasing shame further completes the healing of shame. Releasing means we longer wish to carry the burden of shame nor risk its negative pulls on us once again.

Let's take a look at each of these five elements in detail and their application to codependency and self-recovery.

- **Recognize and understand your shame triggers:** In your study of emotional awareness and expression, you learned to recognize and name your feelings. The same is true for recognizing and naming shame. Sometimes shame is a deeper feeling hidden by anger, embarrassment, or shyness. Perhaps you can already identify your shame triggers. It's okay if you don't know them by name yet. Here are some questions for you to think about before we talk further:

  - Are you aware when you feel shame?

    » Where do you feel shame in your body?

    » What specific feelings arise in you that let you know you feel shame?

    » What thoughts alert you to your shame?

  - Are you aware of things you feel ashamed of? (There is no need to name them right now. We are just working on awareness.)

  - Do you have any particular things you do when you feel ashamed?

- **Develop critical awareness about your shame and its sources:** Critical awareness involves understanding the sources, accuracy, and impact of what you have become aware of. Seeing the reality of self, others, and your situations has been a theme in your self-recovery work already. It appears again here to help you transform shame from an amorphous dark weight within you to self-compassion and the opportunity for change. These questions, modified from Brown's exercises, may help you better understand your sources of shame:

  - How do you want people to perceive you?

    » Why is this perception important to you?

    » Where did you learn to value this perception? Consider the circles of influence on self-development to explore your sources.

  - How do you *not* want to be perceived?

    » Why is this perception unattractive to you?

    » Where does this belief come from? Again, consider the circles of influence on self-development to explore your sources.

  - Do external expectations that you cannot, do not, or will not meet cause you shame?

  - Have any situations in your life caused you shame?

  As you increase your awareness, the facts will help you see that your shame may be based on unrealistic or unfair expectations, the actions of others, and things beyond your control. Such realizations can give you a fresh, realistic perspective on your shame, and you can be more compassionate with your self and open to the next three elements of transforming shame.

- **Become willing to reach out to safe others:** You learned that willingness is an essential ingredient of change. Willingness comes from within. It involves something you want to do and are ready to do. In this case, you are willing to reach out to safe others. Reaching out may be scary for you. Shame itself makes reaching out difficult, and often codependency can make you reluctant to ask for help. Reaching out to safe others becomes possible as you understand your shame better. Safe others are people who understand you and support your self-recovery work. They believe in you and wish you well. They will not make you sorry you told them something about you.

  - Who in your life is a safe person to reach out to?

  - Who in your life cares about you and wishes you well?

  - Can you imagine reaching out to them?

Remember that I, too, can be your safe person, and our therapy sessions will always be a safe place where you can reach out for help.

- **Speak to safe others about your shame:** When you are ready, you can talk with this safe other person about your shame, your experiences with it, and what you understand about it. If you are speaking with a person who is fully present and engaged with you, you will feel the empathy they have for you. This empathy builds connection, which helps you realize you are not alone, not unusual, and not broken. You have transformed your shame into feeling accepted, affirmed, and of value.

- **Release your shame:** Trauma specialist Frank Anderson (2023) teaches that releasing your shame is an important next step in the healing process. As you feel that your shame wounds are healed, having a way to release the artifacts of your shame offers you additional healing. **Client Worksheet 16: Releasing** can help you create letting-go strategies to use when you are ready to detach the weight upon you, which is not yours to carry and does not serve you.

Releasing

Study

When you feel ready, releasing a feeling, expectation, disappointment, worry, or wish can be helpful to your healing. Instead of letting old issues reignite (which is not unusual), you can create a letting-go strategy that feels right to you. Here are some ideas for releasing:

- Write down what you wish to release. Then:
  - Destroy what you've written by burning it, dissolving it, or tearing it up
  - Put what you've written in a public mailbox with no address or return address
- Understand what troubles you in an accurate, new way and adopt that view
- In your mind's eye, figuratively hand back harmful messages to the people who gave them to you
- Connect with your spiritual beliefs and hand off, place, give, or entrust to them whatever you wish to release
- Say to your self:
  - *Not mine*
  - *Not true*
  - *No place for this idea or message in my life*
- Release through your exhalations
- Use movement to shake off, cast away, or melt away
- Let go in an imagined or physical way to the elements: wind, fire, air, water
- Forgive self or others

Self-Reflection

Do any of these ideas appeal to you? If yes, which ones?

_____

_____

Can you think of any of your own of ways to let go?

_____

_____

This Week

This week, identify something you feel ready to release. Perhaps it is an old feeling or a persistent worry that you have healed as best as you can. Maybe it is an aspect of your shame you have been working on. Then practice releasing it, using one of the letting-go strategies that appeals to you.

What did you release and how?

_____

_____

Did any feelings or parts show up as you let go?

_____

_____

Are there any feelings or parts you are aware of now?

_____

_____

Notes to Self

_____

_____

_____

_____

Strategy 51

Learn **guilt management**.

As mentioned earlier, shame and guilt often travel with codependency. Again, shame is a feeling that something is wrong with you, while guilt is the feeling that you have done something wrong. While guilt may seem less severe than shame, it can be easy for codependent individuals to lose self when they feel guilty.

In my clinical experience, helping clients manage their guilt is essential to their self-recovery growth. I commonly find that as a client is progressing in knowing self and finding their voice, guilt enters their work: "Yes, but I feel guilty about that" or "I would feel too guilty if I said that." Guilt can easily overpower other thoughts and feelings, keeping clients stuck in their same patterns of overfunctioning for others and underfunctioning for self. Helping them to address guilt in an accurate way and learn to manage this powerful feeling is foundational to deeper changes.

Accuracy about guilt means discerning whether the guilt is merited or not. Sometimes we feel guilty because we really have done something wrong: we said something we regret, we did not tell the truth, we did not come through for someone who was counting on us. This type of guilt, known as *merited guilt*, can be healthy and motivating. "Healthy" means we recognize that we have done something that does not match our values. "Motivating" means it creates energy within us for repair. The twelve-step fellowships speak of "making amends," which goes beyond an apology—instead, we plan how we can change our behaviors so as to not do that wrong thing again.

Unmerited guilt means we feel badly even though we have not done anything wrong. Yes, that sounds like shame, and let's says we are quite close to where shame and guilt hold hands. But to give our clients more resources for guilt, let's study what unmerited guilt looks like in the codependent client and what they can do to manage this guilt. **Handout 21: Guilt and Codependency** can help with this. Building from the work of Melanie Greenberg (2016), the list encourages your client to develop a more accurate, appreciative perspective on self and guilt-producing situations and offers ideas for managing guilt.

Guilt and Codependency

Guilt shows up with codependency in a number of ways, even when you have not done anything wrong. You may feel guilty when you:

- Say "no" to someone

- Believe you have disappointed or displeased someone

- Have your own needs and preferences that are different from others

- Take time for your self

- Receive help from someone

- Feel bad about feeling guilty

Here are some suggestions to help you work with your guilty parts so you don't lose your self in your guilt but instead have more space to listen and attend to you.

- **Recognize what you *have* done:** Codependent people often feel like they have not done enough, that they should respond to all requests of them, or that they do not want to displease or disappoint others. When you feel this way, take time to write down all the things you *have* done for the person you are concerned about. This list is for your benefit, to help you keep a more balanced view of your offerings to others. Really take in this accurate data: does whatever you haven't done truly outweigh all that you *have* done?

- **Appreciate what you *have* done:** As you absorb the content of your list, see if you can appreciate all you have done for this person and for others. You're not giving out awards here, but you are taking time to honestly recognize and value what you have done.

- **Be careful of all-or-nothing thinking:** Many people, codependent people in particular, think in terms of all or nothing, right or wrong, me or nobody. Learning to live in the gray, as opposed to black or white, is a sign of mental health. This means believing and saying, "Sometimes I can do that. Sometimes I can't." "I am available some of the time, but not all of the time." "I know some of the answers, but not all the answers."

- **Be aware of other feelings you may also be experiencing:** Guilt can be so strong that it drowns out your awareness of other emotions going on at the same time. Pause and see if you notice additional emotions about whatever has you feeling guilty—these may range from relief to anger, from excitement to irritation. Allowing these other emotions to be heard counterbalances the power of guilt. Spend time with these other emotions. They have much to tell you about the choices you are making for you.

- **Re-mind your self of why you said no:** Many times, as soon as we deliver our no, guilt starts moving in. Often, we join the guilt rather than stay anchored with our solid reasons for saying no. Remember your reasons and re-mind your self of them. I like to hyphenate the word—*re-mind*—to emphasize that you are re-setting your mind. As your guilt settles in, so do your errors in thinking. Rather than join those thought distortions that support your guilt, you want to intentionally change your thinking to include the full and accurate picture of what you feel guilty about.

- **Re-mind your self that it is okay *and* important to take care of your own needs:** When your thoughts begin feeding your guilt and your mind is softening on your "no," re-mind your self as often as necessary of the reasons why it's okay and important to take care of you.

Cynthia, Shame, and Guilt

Let's return to Cynthia, the 50-year-old mother suffering from exhaustion, confusion, and fear as she tried to help her adult daughter, Jenna, who was in alcohol recovery.

Cynthia made the decision to stay in counseling for a while. She said she did not know what else to do to get out of her ruts of caregiving and worry. She became a motivated client whose therapy goals included learning to set boundaries with her daughter. She explained that she wanted to help Jenna and she wanted her own life too, though she had no idea what that might look like.

To address her goal, we began work with the material in self-competence with confidence. We first worked on the five foundational skills. Cynthia was very glad to learn that she did not have to act immediately on her daughter's requests. The notion of checking in with herself first was foreign yet appealing. It was also scary. She learned to pause, connect with her breath, quiet her thoughts, and release tension from her body. She especially liked to use her senses to come into the present moment so she could think better.

Cynthia had always felt ashamed of her daughter's problems. Shame had kept Cynthia from spending time with family and friends who might ask about Jenna and have opinions about what Cynthia should do. "What kind of person is ashamed of their child?" she asked. However, Cynthia said she felt so much better when she was able to tell me about her shame. She had never spoken with anyone about it in the honest way she was able to with me. This transformed Cynthia's shame, lightened her emotional burden, and freed her to talk more honestly and realistically about herself and her situations.

Guilt management was quite difficult for Cynthia, who called herself the Queen of Guilt. She felt resigned to feeling guilty about most everything. I introduced the idea that she could learn ways to avoid joining her guilt. She was curious and willing to try to understand this.

Situation by situation, Cynthia learned to figure out whether her guilt was merited or not. If it was merited, she usually apologized and did something to fix the situation. If her guilt was unmerited, Cynthia learned to recognize and appreciate what she had done for her daughter, re-mind her self of why she said no to her daughter's request, and re-mind her self that it was okay and important to also consider her own needs and preferences. Cynthia's intentional practice of these new skills helped her become better able to quiet her guilt and stick with her nos.

Strategy 52

Learn **assertiveness**.

I have been teaching assertiveness as a life skill for 40 years. Early in my counseling career, I developed a continuum to teach assertiveness to the teenagers I worked with at a juvenile corrections facility. Over the decades since then, I have frequently used that continuum with a variety of clients who needed guidance in speaking up for self. Many of us don't know this basic skill. Instead, we are passive and don't say what is true for us, or we get upset and act and speak in aggressive ways. Codependent people, in particular, can have difficulty with self-expression. Worried they may upset someone, they do not speak up until, frustrated with always being the go-to person, they can explode.

This continuum between passive and aggressive behaviors is demonstrated in **Handout 22: Assertiveness Training**. You can use the following script when introducing the handout.

Psychoeducation Script
Assertiveness Training

This is a diagram to help you learn assertiveness. At the top of the illustration, you'll see that the behaviors we are studying range from passive through assertive to aggressive. You can fall anywhere on this continuum at any point in your interactions with others. The goals of this assertiveness training are to increase your skills in expressing your self assertively and to develop your ability to regulate your self along the continuum with assertiveness as your intention.

The illustration has three categories of information listed under each expressive style: the first row is a description of that style, the second row describes how emotions are involved, and the third row shows how respect is conveyed.

Let's look at the descriptions of each style. First, let's consider passive.

> [**Note to Clinician:** Present and discuss the handout's content listed under *passive*.]

Now let's go to the other end of the continuum and study aggressive.

> [**Note to Clinician:** Present and discuss the handout's content listed under *aggressive*.]

Now let's look at assertive in the center. Assertiveness is about being anchored in your "I" statement. When we are assertive, we are speaking for self. We have thought ahead and know what is true for us, and we express it by starting our sentence with "I." This is an excellent setup for clearly communicating for self: "I [fill in the blank.]"

Sometimes it takes time and effort to figure out your "I" statement, but it is there waiting for you to recognize it. As you make your "I" statement, you do not have to defend it or over-explain it. It is perfectly okay for you to have your own thoughts, feelings, and needs and to express them in simple

---

and solid ways. If someone pushes back on your "I" statement, be ready to act like a broken record with clear and committed repetitions of your "I" statement.

[**Note to Clinician:** Review and discuss the handout's content listed under *assertive*.]

As you stay steady with your assertive response, you are also paying attention to any temptations to move on the continuum toward passive or aggressive. It's normal if you feel pulled one way or the other, or both. Re-anchor in your "I" statement as often as needed. Assertiveness is not necessarily easy, but it is worth the effort.

The second row in the chart looks at emotional expression. When you are able to stay in the assertive zone, you are aware of and in control of your emotions. They are expressed through your clear "I" statement: "I don't want to do that now." "I can help you on Saturday." "I feel hurt by what you said." If you move toward passivity, you may start stuffing down or ignoring your emotions. If you move toward aggression, you may not be aware of or in control of your emotions and weaponize them to overpower or hurt the other person.

The third line of the illustration is about respect. When you are assertive—centered, clear, and steady—you show a great deal of respect for your self and the other person. There is no attacking or abandoning of your self or others. You are not saying or suppressing things you will later regret. When you become too passive or aggressive, respect for self and others diminishes. This is where habitual patterns of arguing, submission, or resentment can take hold.

Knowing how to express your self assertively is an important piece in your self-recovery work. Developing your assertive voice helps you become responsive, not reactive, toward self and to others.

Is there an "I" statement you would like to work on with me today? We can start by identifying something you would like to assertively say to someone in your life. Then you can practice your assertiveness here with me using some of the ideas on the handout.

Assertiveness Training*

Continuum of Expressive Behaviors

PASSIVE	ASSERTIVE	AGGRESSIVE
You may: • Withdraw • Avoid • Hide • Remain silent • Go along	• You use "I" statements to clearly express your feelings, needs, or thoughts. • You do not need to use elaborate justifications or explanations. • You use the "broken record"—a repetition of your "I" statements when confronted with invitations or attacks to move you from your stated position.	You may: • Use "you" statements • Demean • Accuse • Blame • Act pushy, forceful • Threaten • Attack others verbally or physically
• Your emotions are ignored or not acknowledged.	• You remain aware of your emotions and they are under your control.	• Your are unaware of your emotions or they are out of your control.
• Your behavior shows no respect for your self or others.	• Your behavior shows respect for your self and others.	• Your behavior shows no respect for your self and others.

---

* Adapted from *Disentangle: When You've Lost Your Self in Someone Else* (2nd ed., p. 253), by N. L. Johnston, 2020, Central Recovery Press.

Strategy 53

Learn **boundary setting**.

In my early clinical work with codependency during the late 1990s, I created counseling groups that brought together a variety of clients, all with the core issue of loss of self in others. As these clients worked toward developing a healthy self separate from and simultaneously in relationship with others, their need for boundaries became clear.

Setting boundaries does not mean establishing walls that cut you off from others or becoming rigidly attached to rules and procedures that don't necessarily work in all situations. Instead, setting boundaries means defining limits of what you will and won't tolerate in a particular situation. Setting boundaries means you are able to listen to your self, know your limits, and firmly assert those limits to your self and the people they may involve.

Setting boundaries is a healthy thing to do. It helps us know the parameters of our relationships and interactions. Our children need boundaries; so do the adults with whom we interact. We even need to set limits with our self. The boundary-setting skills taught in this strategy can be applied in any of these situations.

Boundary setting is particularly important in our work with codependent clients. Many a codependent person will tell you they are not good at setting boundaries. Either they just don't set them, or they give in or back down from boundaries they set. No blame here—this is part of the codependent client's challenge. Here are some voices from clients on this topic:

- "If I say no, they won't call me again."

- "If I ask for too much, they will leave me."

- "If I am not available then, they will think badly of me."

- "If I can only help them for two hours, they will think I don't like them."

- "If I can't complete the assignment until Friday, they will think I am lazy."

- "If I say I won't pay for that, they will be mad at me."

- "If I take time to walk each day, I look selfish."

Often the need for boundaries appears in the middle of some upset, fight, disappointment, or worry. If we are not mindful, we can blurt out a boundary that is not true for us or one that we are not ready to live with: "Get out." "I want a divorce." "You can't go to the prom." "You can't ever _____ again." We react instead of respond.

Learning how to set boundaries is a new assignment for your codependent client. Learning to assert and live with those boundaries is an even greater challenge, as those actions tap into deep codependent fears of abandonment, displeasure, conflict, and loss of control. For this reason, I teach boundary setting in three thoughtful, focused parts:

1. Discerning your boundary

2. Expressing your boundary

3. Living with your boundary

As relationship therapist Nedra Glover Tawwab (2023) says, our clients are playing out old patterns, and we need to teach them ways to act differently. **Handout 23: Setting Healthy Boundaries** walks you and your client through important skills that can help them become more effective in boundary setting and, in fact, establish new ways of being with self and with others.

Healthy Boundary Setting

1) Discerning Your Boundary

Boundary setting begins with you. Step aside and take time to check in with you. Figure out what limit is true for you and what boundaries you have within your control. Here are some guidelines for tuning into your self and discerning your boundary:

- **Slow down:** Before you try to set a limit that is true for you and is one you can live with, pause, take a breath, take a break, and connect with you.

- **Listen to you:** You may hear the voice of the other person strongly and clearly in your mind. Now is the time to quiet their voice and listen to your four areas of self: body, mind, emotions, and spirit. Each area has valuable information for you about the boundary that is right for you. Listen to all four areas. Your mind may be telling you one thing and your body may be giving you a different message. It is important to listen to and respect all these internal messages as you decide.

- **Find your "I" statement:** After listening to these areas of your self and weighing the perhaps conflicting internal messages of yes and no, create a statement that begins with "I" to express the boundary you are deciding on. For example: "I cannot afford to do that" or "I can give you two hours each week to work on that."

  - **Express it as a statement, not a question:** Questions are tentative and invite collaboration: "Would it be okay with you if I _____?" A statement has strength and clarity: "I have decided that I will not be able to _____." You can do this!

  - **Edit your "I" statement:** Make sure your boundary is what you mean and that you can and will live with it.

  - **Rehearse your "I" statement with a safe person:** Say your boundary out loud to your self and to someone who is supporting you in your growth.

> ### Into Action
> #### You and Discerning Your Boundary
>
> Think of something going on in your life where boundary setting is needed. Is there a boundary you would like to set with your self or with someone else?
>
> Working with this situation, apply the steps we just studied in part one.

2) Expressing Your Boundary Assertively

These skills help you express your boundary to the person it involves. Whether that person is you or another person in your life, these suggestions are designed to help you stay connected with self and steady with your well-discerned boundary as you deliver it:

- **State your boundary assertively:** The assertiveness skills you learned in the previous strategy come directly into play here. Stay centered in your "I" statement and be ready to repeat it, as you may feel challenged by the other person or by your own feelings of fear, worry, or mistrust of self. Be aware of your tone and speak in a neutral, informing way. The following recommendations will also help you stay in the zone of assertiveness.

- **Be prepared to stick with your boundary:** It is important that the boundary you have set is one you really mean and can live with. Finding the boundary you can commit to is part of discerning. As you tell it to the other person, stay connected with your commitment. Changing or letting go of your boundary suggests that you can be persuaded to step down from something important to you.

- **Don't over-explain your reasons for your boundary:** Codependent people can feel like they have to fully explain and justify what they assert for self. Over-explaining can get you into trouble. It opens conversations further and can seem to be inviting negotiations or other solutions that do not match the boundary you are setting. Instead of explaining, say things once, maybe twice if needed. Granted, sometimes clarification may be needed, or the boundary may need to be reinforced through repetition (similar to the "broken record" technique discussed in Handout 22). But after that, be careful of your impulses to explain or defend the boundary you are setting. Saying what you need to say and then stopping shows strength and resolution.

- **Stick with the specific topic:** When we are upset or nervous, we can get off the topic at hand. When you express your boundary, stay focused on your "I" statement and the specific situation it is addressing. Notice when you feel drawn into talking about past issues or other complaints, and redirect you back to your well-discerned boundary.

- **Stay in the present:** This suggestion reinforces your efforts to stick with the specific topic. Being present with self, the other person, and your boundary can be centering and empowering. Use your breath and body to anchor you as you engage in this boundary-setting situation.

Into Action
You and Expressing Your Boundary Assertively

Let's walk through applying each of the suggestions in part 2 to the boundary you discerned in part 1.

First, let's talk about the suggestions. Which ones appeal to you? What are your challenges to expressing your boundary?

Now, if you are willing, we can role-play expressing your boundary. First, I will play you and model the skills you are learning. You will play the other person. That helps me to know what you expect they will say and do as you express your boundary, and I can teach you additional responses to help you stay centered and clear.

Then we will reverse the roles and you will get to practice expressing your boundary.

3) Living with Your Boundary

Living with your boundary is an inside job. Once you have discerned and expressed your boundary, you have the opportunity to live with your boundary. If the boundary is one you have set with your self, you are now poised to make the change you want for you. If your boundary is with someone else, you may well be adjusting to changes in your relationship with them as a result of your boundary. Here are some ideas to help you along the way:

- **Re-mind your self of the reasons for your boundary:** Remember the action of "re-minding" that we studied in managing guilt? In the case of boundary setting, re-minding is re-setting our thoughts so we remember *why* we are setting our boundary. As time goes by and emotions calm down, it is easy to let go of a boundary. We forget what prompted the boundary and why it was important to us then. If we don't re-mind our self why we set a boundary and choose to let it go, the need for it very often shows up again.

- **Connect with your strengths and belief in self:** Tawwab (2023) conveys this beautifully to her clients: "You can do this!" "You've got this!" "I think you have more power than you think." "I think you can be courageous." Such wonderful messages invite you to connect with your strengths. In the middle of strong emotions and relationship upsets, we all lose track of our strengths. Now is a good time to reconnect with and discover even more strengths within.

- **Listen, but be careful not to over-defend or over-explain your choices:** Self-recovery is not selfish. We are strengthening self so we can live and love in more mutual ways. When you set a boundary, you can listen to what the other person has to say and let them know what you hear from them. At the same time, stay connected with you and your boundary. Don't try to get them to agree with you or be pleased with your boundary. Such efforts to convince the other person can entangle you all over again.

- **Know when to stop participating in a conversation about your boundary:** There is definitely an art to knowing when to stop a conversation. Stopping at the right time increases the chance of keeping our center, making our point, and ending the conversation in a healthy way. When you tune in to your four areas of self as well as the tone and direction of the conversation, you know when it is time to stop talking.

- **Stop:** We sometimes know that we need to stop talking, yet we still don't. Stopping our self and stepping away is a crucial skill to develop. We can save our self and the interaction if we assertively say what we want to say, talk about it with centeredness, tune in to when it's time to stop, and then stop.

Into Action
You and Living with Your Boundary

Look at each suggestion in part 3 and see how it applies to you and the boundary you want to set from parts 1 and 2.

What can help you to remember why you set your boundary?

What are some of your strengths that can help you with boundary setting?

What tools can help you listen to someone else and stay connected with self at the same time?

When do you think you should stop participating in a conversation? What are the cues within you that warn you of this—do you sense any particular thoughts, feelings, or body responses?

What can you do to stop participating in a conversation that is becoming problematic?

Cynthia, Assertiveness, and Boundaries

Cynthia and I continued to work through the skill sets in self-competence with confidence. Cynthia felt strongly about her counseling goal of learning to set healthy boundaries, so we continued to build her self-foundation for boundary setting by practicing the five foundational skills.

- *Assertiveness Training: Cynthia was quite enthusiastic about learning to be assertive. She had never thought about using an "I" statement—to her, that seemed like a selfish thing to do. Codependent individuals are so used to talking about someone else that this shift to "I" is profound. As with her work on guilt management, Cynthia had to bring awareness and intention in order to shift her focus to self and to assert what she wanted for self, even with me.*

- *Healthy Boundary Setting: Learning to transform shame, manage guilt, and speak assertively prepared Cynthia for the three parts of boundary setting:*

  - *Part 1: Discerning Your Boundary: Cynthia learned to first step away from her daughter's problem or request and listen to self. She would use any or all of the five foundational skills to ground herself. Then she would ask herself, "What can I honestly offer to Jenna's request? What can I offer that considers my needs and resources as well?" Cynthia's connection with self helped her construct her solid "I" statement instead of reactively making an offer she did not want to make or exploding with anger yet still saying yes.*

  - *Part 2: Expressing Your Boundary: With her guilt management and assertiveness skills in hand, Cynthia was able to state her "I" statement in amazing new ways. She was careful not to elaborate too much about her boundary or defend it. A solid, clear answer reflected the strength she was building for self: "No. I cannot give you more money." "I am available until noon if you need a ride." "I will be out this evening."*

  - *Part 3: Living with Your Boundary: Though this part was a challenge for Cynthia, she was committed to making these changes for self. She was particularly helped by reminding her self of why she was setting the boundary. (She was also surprised at how often she needed to do that.) Cynthia became more aware and accepting of saying no, and she worked hard to stop herself from engaging further in conversations with Jenna when she knew more talk would not serve either of them well.*

Insights and Intentions

Consider the strategies introduced in this chapter:

49. Practice **five foundational skills**.

50. Learn to **transform shame**.

51. Learn **guilt management**.

52. Learn **assertiveness**.

53. Learn **boundary setting**.

What have you learned in this chapter about helping your client develop self-competence *with increasing confidence*?

_____

_____

Which handouts, worksheets, or scripts in this chapter seem particularly useful in your work with codependent clients?

_____

_____

Have you identified any skill sets you may want to develop in order to balance self and others, such as guilt management or boundary setting?

_____

_____

Are there handouts, worksheets, or scripts from this chapter you might intentionally bring to your practice or apply in your own life?

_____

_____

CHAPTER 9

Self-Attunement
Established with Care

The first three elements of self-recovery—self-understanding, self-awareness, and self-competence—are all essential to making the shift to a healthy internal focus, but self-attunement is the element that solidifies your client's genuine, reliable connection with self. Self-attunement completes the circle of four interlocking elements that hold and support the relationship-with-self in the center by adding intention, commitment, comfort, and security to your client's evolving relationship-with-self.

Developed from attachment theory, self-attunement acknowledges ways that codependency reflects insecure attachment styles. As we move through this chapter, you will understand the meaning of self-attunement and learn self-attunement exercises that will help your client identify desired qualities for their relationship-with-self, learn to access self, and cultivate paths to their relationship-with-self.

Strategy 54

Understand **self-attunement**.

There are two areas of developmental study that contribute to the concept of self-attunement. The first area of study is the work of Alice Miller (1981), who explains in *The Drama of the Gifted Child* that a person's *true self* may be split off from them because their primary caregivers were not able to or did not attune to their feelings and needs as an infant. The caregivers did not mirror or echo what the infant was conveying to them. Instead, the caregivers needed or allowed the child to satisfy their own needs. As a result, the child learned to attune to the well-being of their parents and developed a false self, a self not connected with or free to be the person they are.

Attachment theory is the second area of developmental study supporting self-attunement. As we move through this strategy, recall our previous discussion of attachment styles and their relationship to codependency with an emphasis on insecure attachment styles—avoidant and ambivalent. Next, we will look carefully at the qualities that foster a *secure* attachment style.

An infant becomes securely attached to a caregiver who is sensitive, warm, and responsive to their needs on a consistent basis (Bowlsby, 1988). A secure attachment style is characterized by the child's use of the caregiver as a trustworthy and secure base from which to explore and master the world. This creates an internal security that gives the child confidence, comfort, and the ability to grow (Ainsworth & Bell, 1970; Ainsworth et al., 1979/2015).

Though we wish it were not so, many of us were raised in ways that did not let us connect with our true self. Trauma and abuse denied self, as did parenting styles based on patriarchy and authoritarianism. Self-consideration may have been unacceptable in an individual's social, cultural, political, and religious worlds. For any or all of these reasons, a secure attachment style was not possible.

If this is so, the recovery of self starts with awareness and understanding of our developmental experiences and resulting attachment styles. For those with insecure attachment styles, the grief process sets in almost immediately. Our loss and sadness about what we did not receive as we grew up naturally appears, along with other feelings including anger and what-ifs. This is when we can use the material in strategy 40 (p. 122) for authentic healing from grief.

From there, we can go further by establishing a relationship-with-self that offers what we did *not* receive from our relationships with our primary caregivers—sensitivity, responsiveness, consistency, warmth, trustworthiness, security, comfort, and the ability to grow, among other things. The growth in our relationship-with-self is fostered by self-attunement—that is, attuning to our body, mind, emotions, and spirit, hearing these areas of self correctly, and making adjustments that improve the tone and quality of our life.

Our relationship-with-self is ultimately about becoming our own parent, therapist, teacher, and friend. When we previously discussed emotional awareness and expression, I cited Nhất Hạnh's (1991) suggestion to look deeply into the causes and nature of feelings as the fifth and final step in transforming feelings. He describes this exploration as being like psychotherapy. Nhất Hạnh says that the ultimate intention for the patient in psychotherapy is to connect with their own internal psychotherapist, who is available to them at all times.

Similarly, Miller (1981) describes a psychotherapeutic course of integration, which helps the client know and be their true self. The course first involves accessing and expressing feelings within the therapy sessions. Then, through their emotional awareness and the therapeutic relationship with their therapist, the client is able to experience, express, and process feelings from childhood long hidden from self. Miller explains that the client is able to separate from the therapist once they have reliably mourned and can handle their childhood feelings on their own. In essence, their relationship with their true self is now established, and they can foster this relationship on their own.

The thought of establishing this relationship-with-self can be disappointing for our clients at first—they deeply desire a secure attachment with *another human being*. That may well become possible, but it is essential for them to first grieve what they longed for and did not experience. When they are ready to learn how to give those very wished-for things to self, they can have a secure base within themselves that allows them to develop healthy relationships with others.

Strategy 55

Identify **desired qualities** of a relationship-with-self.

The material in the previous strategy was essentially for you, the clinician, to familiarize you with this concept of self-attunement and its role in self-recovery. Now it's time to invite your client into this work. We will use **Handout 24: Self-Attunement and Establishing Your Relationship-with-Self** and **Client Worksheet 17: Qualities of Your Relationship-with-Self** to educate and engage them in this process of self-attunement and to consider the qualities they desire for their relationship-with-self.

Self-Attunement and Establishing Your Relationship-with-Self

Let's begin to establish your relationship-with-self. Yes, that's a thing. You can have a relationship with your self just like you have a relationship with your family members and friends. In fact, having a relationship-with-self is what will help you pull all of your self-recovery work together.

You have learned about self-understanding, self-awareness, and self-competence. The hope is that those three elements of self-recovery are helping you consider your own feelings and needs more, and you are better able to balance care of self and others. Now we are adding the fourth element, self-attunement, to solidify your recovery from codependency. Self-attunement adds spark and commitment to your budding relationship-with-self and supports your work with the other three elements.

This idea of self-attunement comes from attachment theory and the concept of true self versus false self:

Alice Miller (1981) explains that a person's true self may be split off from them because their primary caregivers were not able to or did not attune to their feelings and needs as an infant. The caregiver did not mirror or echo what the infant was conveying to them. The caregiver instead needed or allowed the child to satisfy their own needs. As a result, the child learned to attune to the well-being of their parent and developed a false self, a self not connected with or free to be the person they are.

Attachment theorists describe a secure attachment style in this way: A secure attachment is characterized by the child's use of the caregiver as a secure base from which to explore and master the world. The caregiver has offered sensitivity, warmth, and consistency to the child. The child has learned the parent is caring, trustworthy, and responsive and provides a safe haven for them. This creates an internal security that gives the child confidence, comfort, and the ability to grow (Bowlby, 1988; Ainsworth & Bell, 1970; Ainsworth et al., 1979/2015).

Drawing from key words in the description of true self and secure attachment, self-attunement invites you to offer your self these fundamental qualities that promote your internal security and growth:

- Attuned
- Sensitive
- Responsive
- Consistent
- Warm
- Caring
- Trustworthy
- Confident
- Comfortable
- Safe haven

Qualities of Your Relationship-with-Self

Study

Handout 24: Self-Attunement and Establishing Your Relationship-with-Self is full of information about self-attunement, the fourth element of self-recovery. Read it and take time to absorb the qualities that foster a secure relationship with your true self.

Now, write your own list of qualities you appreciate in an important relationship in your life. This could be with a parent, another family member, your children, or a friend. Identify what qualities of that relationship allow you to feel safe and free to be your authentic self with that person.

_____

_____

Self-Reflection

How do you feel about this idea of a relationship-with-self? Does it appeal to you? Can you imagine having such a relationship? Do you already have one?

_____

_____

How willing are you to develop your relationship-with-self?

_____

_____

What would help you develop your relationship-with-self?

_____

_____

Looking at **handout 24**'s list of qualities that foster a secure relationship with your true self, which of these qualities do you want to offer your self? Pick as many as you wish.

_____

_____

Looking at your list of qualities that you appreciate in your relationships, which qualities would you especially like to offer to your self? Pick as many as you wish.

_____

_____

This Week

This week keep in mind the qualities you would like for your relationship-with-self.

Notice what you are offering to your relationship with you.

Are you remembering your relationship-with-self?

_____

_____

Are you offering the desired relationship qualities you put on your list? Which ones?

_____

_____

If you are not offering your desired qualities, how are you treating your relationship-with-self? What messages are you giving to you?

_____

_____

Would you like to improve the tone and messaging you bring to your relationship with you? How might you do this?

_____

_____

Strategy 56

Learn to **access** self.

This entire workbook is about helping your client access self. It is the core shift in self-recovery that gives your codependent client the ability to change from their habitually dominant other-centeredness to a healthy consideration of self and others.

So why have a specific strategy here for accessing self?

The reason is that learning to attune to self and then building a relationship-with-self invites more intentional awareness, discernment, and care than ever before. Your client can learn about self, become more aware of self, and develop new skills without developing a relationship-with-self. Similarly, in raising a child, we can provide for them, protect them, and teach them, all without having a relationship with them. So much more is possible, however, when an authentic relationship takes hold. Self-attunement is about doing just that for and with our self.

The next two strategies are designed to help your client deepen their access to self. Each strategy will include an experiential exercise to help them with their work.

Strategy 57

Sustain a healthy **internal focus**.

Developing and sustaining an internal focus requires intention and practice. **Self-Attunement Exercise 1: Fostering Your Internal Connections through Conscious Awareness** offers fundamental reminders and practices that can help your client access self when they feel safe and ready. The exercise is best used by guiding the client through it. As the client completes the exercise, invite them to become aware of things that are true for them but not listed. This encourages them yet again to connect with self.

Fostering Your Internal Connections through Conscious Awareness

- Pause periodically throughout your day in a safe place.

- Notice what you are paying attention to and are perhaps lost in:

    – Thoughts _____

    – Feelings _____

    – Body sensations _____

    – Regrets _____

    – Future plans _____

    – Worries, fears _____

    – Demands, expectations, disappointments _____

    – Hopes, dreams, wishes _____

    – Relationship issues _____

    – _____

    – _____

- Perhaps some part of you is front and center: _____

- Now, gently bring your self into the present moment through any or all of these techniques. You may have some techniques of your own to add to your list:

    – Use of your senses

    – Connecting with your diaphragmatic breath

    – Brief body scan from head to toe

    – _____

    – _____

- Spend five minutes practicing whatever helps you dwell in the present moment. Be patient as you learn this new skill of pausing and connecting with you. Your thoughts may jump in. When they do, simply notice them and return your focus to your breath, body, or sense.

- Now, with your grounded awareness of self, check in with your four areas of self: body, mind, emotions, and spirit. Notice without judgment. This is just about paying attention in a full and balanced way to what is within you.

- When you are ready, let go of your noticing and simply follow your diaphragmatic breath for several more cycles. Scan your body from head to toe as you breathe and release tension. This can feel like a gentle, cleansing waterfall over and through you.

Strategy 58

Meet their **gatekeepers**.

The gatekeepers are who we run into as we are trying to connect with self. As your client settles into calm and awareness, it is quite likely that various gatekeepers meet them at the entrance to their garden of self within.

There are all types of gardens. There are vegetable gardens, rock gardens, wooded gardens, and combinations of these. Gardens can be located in your backyard, on a shoreline, on a mountaintop, on an empty city lot, on your patio, or by a window in your house. Gardens can be planted in the earth, in fancy pots, or in recycled cans. You get the point. Gardens can be as different as we are as people. But in this book, *garden* does not necessarily mean a floral garden with birds singing. The "garden of self" is instead a rich metaphor for the cultivation of self. This metaphor highlights the planting and tending that both a garden and the self require for healthy growth.

Gardens need lots of attending and responding to. The basics of sun and water are essential to a successful garden, as are fertilization, pruning, and harvesting. Similarly, the growth of our relationship-with-self is dependent on providing self with our health essentials as well as regular nurturing care.

Many gardens have fences and gates to protect the plants and the land. Garden gates can be a beautiful piece of art; they can also be functional. Whatever the gate's form, it is there for necessary protection for the garden's growth. In the same way, we have our gatekeepers at the entrance to our garden of self. They greet us at the gate as we slow down and start to access self. We will need to stop, greet, and meet them in order to safely and fully enter our garden of self.

Meeting the gatekeepers involves returning to the work on parts of self we studied in **Handout 12: Parts and Self-Recovery** (p. 116). This passage from that handout reflects how self-recovery not only builds on itself but also circles back and enriches what was learned before:

Self-recovery is about ultimately developing a relationship-with-self. This involves getting to know the different parts of self. We each have a variety of parts in us, and we often think and speak about them very naturally—for example, "Part of me wants to go out tonight, but another part just wants to stay in." Our parts can serve different roles, and as the parts of self learn to live together in the community of self, an authentic relationship-with-self develops.

That's what self-attunement can foster: an authentic relationship-with-self. In order to self-attune, we must meet, greet, and respond to the gatekeepers who are protecting our garden of self. They mean no harm. In fact, they are there to prevent harm. As we come to know and trust our self, the gatekeepers may not need to be so protective of our access to what is within.

Recognizing these gatekeepers can help your client better understand their difficulties with accessing self, and they will learn what to do when they get to the gate and find that passage into self is protected. After working with **Handout 25: Parts as Gatekeepers**, offer your client **Self-Attunement Exercise 2: Meet, Greet, and Respond to Your Gatekeepers** to practice an interaction with one of their gatekeepers.

Parts as Gatekeepers

Sometimes when we try to quiet our self and look within, all sorts of static shows up in the form of thoughts, feelings, and impulses. Some of that is natural; some of it may be our gatekeepers protecting us from access to what we will call our *garden of self*, a metaphor for our self-growth.

Our gatekeepers are parts of your self that you learned about in **Handout 12: Parts and Self-Recovery**. Read the following list of parts that are especially adept at gatekeeping. Recognizing these parts and being able to name them will be quite helpful as you negotiate access to your garden. And remember, these gatekeepers are protective. While they mean no harm, they may be working too hard to protect you in ways you no longer need.

Protective Gatekeepers

Trauma Responses

- Fight
- Flight
- Freeze
- Fawn
- Fix

Characters

- Inner critic
- Procrastinator
- Shame
- Guilt
- Minimizer
- Resister
- Doubter
- Fear
- Conflict avoider
- "Yes, but . . ."
- Storyteller
- Blamer
- Restless one

Behaviors Associated with Codependency (Yes, behaviors can be gatekeepers, too.)

- Staying busy
- Time for self is a low priority
- Engaging in addictive behaviors
- Blaming others
- Getting stuck in your same patterns or habits

- Reacting, not responding
- Taking care of others
- Living someone else's life
- Scrambling to keep the peace
- Denying self so you won't be abandoned
- Changing your plans to accommodate or please others

Meeting, Greeting, and Responding to Your Gatekeepers

Use this list of suggestions (which build on the list from **handout 12**) when you decide you are ready to meet your gatekeepers:

- Notice the gatekeepers as they present themselves and, if possible, greet them by name.

- Spend time with them and get to know them.

- Quiet your judgment and offer curiosity and patience.

- Ask them about their job and what they are protecting.

- Listen to what they want you to know about them and their work.

- Listen to what they would like from you in the here and now.

- Let them know why you want access within. Tell them what you are up to.

- Let parts help other parts. For example, invite your adult parts to attune to the gatekeepers and respond to them with:

  - Listening
  - Reassurance
  - Patience
  - Protection
  - Care
  - Safety

  - Consistency
  - Wisdom
  - Guidance
  - Consideration
  - Understanding
  - Gratitude

- Ask the gatekeeper: "What will help you feel safe enough for me to enter my garden of self and spend time there?"

- Your goal is to cultivate a reasonable and responsive relationship with your gatekeepers as you would with family, friends, and neighbors.

- As with any authentic relationship, this is an ongoing process, best approached with respect and confidence in your ability to have a good relationship with any and all of your gatekeepers.

Meet, Greet, and Respond to Your Gatekeepers

- Use **Self-Attunement Exercise 1: Fostering Your Internal Connections through Conscious Awareness** to ground and center.

- After five minutes of settling within, *intentionally* visit with your self:

  - First, check in with your four areas of self: body, mind, emotions, and spirit.

  - Do you notice any gatekeepers protecting your access to self? Can you name them?

    _____

    _____

  - Spend some nonjudgmental time with one of your gatekeepers. What is their job? What are they protecting?

    _____

    _____

  - What would this gatekeeper like from you here and now?

    _____

    _____

  - Why do you want access to your garden of self? (Make sure to tell your gatekeeper this answer.)

    _____

    _____

  - What will you do to help your gatekeeper feel safe, allowing them to give you entrance into your garden of self? (Make sure to tell your gatekeeper this answer.)

    _____

    _____

  - Reassure your gatekeeper of your interest and willingness to safely work this out together so you can come and go with their confidence and trust. What can you say to convey this relationship-building message?

    _____

    _____

- If you and you gatekeeper agree on your access to self, thank them and pass through, spending five more minutes simply being with you in calm and stillness.

- If you and your gatekeeper have not yet agreed on your access to self, thank them for their time and protection, and ask if they are willing to talk further at another time. Thank your self for your work as well and exhale fully, releasing whatever energies may have built up in you.

Strategy 59

Cultivate **paths** to their relationship-with-self.

Once we have comfortably gained access to our garden of self, there are paths within to help us find our way to our relationship-with-self. Those paths may not be well-established; it may be hard to see them. This is what your client's work is now about—creating new paths within that help them more easily water, fertilize, and harvest their growing relationship-with-self.

The following three strategies can help clients to establish these paths, or perhaps help them create smaller paths to access their main paths. These strategies include additional self-attunement exercises to help with this internal trailblazing.

Strategy 60

Establish supportive **self-regard**.

Our clients can be so hard on themselves. "That was stupid of me!" "I'll never learn!" "Who would want to be with someone like me?" "I am so mad at myself!" Having repeatedly heard these types of statements from clients, I realized the importance of helping clients become aware of their ingrained belief systems about self, the self-talk they use, and the possibilities of becoming more kind, open, and compassionate with self. Such internal shifts can calm, center, and bring patience to this process of growing self in new ways.

You can use **Self-Attunement Exercise 3: Fostering Your Supportive Self-Regard** to help your client become aware of the messages they give to their self and to invite the possibility of changing their self-talk in the direction of accurate, kind self-support.

Fostering Your Supportive Self-Regard

- Pause periodically throughout your day in a safe place.

- Notice any messages you may be giving to your self. We call this self-talk. Place a check mark by any message you have thought to your self today. Feel free to add any additional ones on the blank lines.

  ❑ "That was stupid of me!"

  ❑ "No one cares what I think."

  ❑ "I don't know what I am doing."

  ❑ "I am hopeless."

  ❑ "What I need is not as important as . . ."

  ❑ "I'll do that for myself later."

  ❑ _____

  ❑ _____

- Pay attention to your messages to you. Do these messages encourage supportive self-regard? Supportive self-regard includes:

  ❑ Being compassionate, kind, and open with self

  ❑ Valuing and trusting self

- Where do you think these messages you are giving your self are coming from?

  _____

  _____

- Would you like to modify your messages to you to be more supportive, kind, or even more accurate? Which messages would promote your self-regard?

  ❑ "I am smart and capable."

  ❑ "I can change and grow."

  ❑ "I have hope."

  ❑ "I can do this."

  ❑ "What I need is important, and I can give that to myself."

  ❑ "I will attend to me first."

  ❑ "I did the best I could, and it was good enough."

  ❑ "I am pleased with . . ."

  ❑ _____

  ❑ _____

- Which messages from the above list could you honestly believe and offer to your self?

  _____

  _____

Strategy 61

Act on things in **their control**.

Ever since the beginning of my self-recovery journey, I have been a fan of the Serenity Prayer as taught in the twelve-step fellowships:

God, grant me the
serenity to accept the things I cannot change, the
courage to change the things I can, and the
wisdom to know the difference.

While the prayer begins with "god," it is more broadly an invitation to tap into our spiritual self as we individually define it. As we live into the prayer, it invites us to lean further into our spirituality to help us let go of what we cannot control as well as to become more adept at controlling what we can.

Codependent clients can be especially challenged by what they can and cannot control. I often explain to my codependent clients, "You are trying to control what you can't, which is the other person, and you are not controlling what you can, which is your self." This is a kind and hopeful correction of how they usually think and operate. Often, without awareness, they are trying to control what they cannot. It is indeed hopeful to become aware of what you *can* do something about.

Controlling behaviors are often associated with codependency. Remember, there is nothing wrong with any behavior associated with codependency up to a point. It's precisely that point that this strategy is focusing on. The prayer asks for "wisdom to know the difference." Helping our clients learn the difference between what they can and cannot control is big. Helping them to have the ability to let go of what they can't control is even bigger.

Handout 26: Acting on Things in Your Control offers details to help your client with each of these three areas of work well described in the prayer: (1) discerning what they can and cannot control (*wisdom*), (2) acting on what they can control (*serenity*), and (3) letting go of what they cannot control (*courage*).

Acting on Things in Your Control

You may be aware of the Serenity Prayer. Often used in the twelve-step programs as a foundation for recovery, it appears in religious circles and well beyond. Self-recovery incorporates it, too.

God grant me the
serenity to accept the things I cannot change, the
courage to change the things I can, and the
wisdom to know the difference

It begins with "god." This is the god of your understanding—in other words, inviting your spirituality into your recovery. You will need the other three areas of self as well—your body, mind, and emotions—to live into the wisdom of this prayer.

Codependency often means trying to control what you can't, which is someone else, while not controlling what you can, which is you. This is good to know. Putting your energy into what you have control over can be powerful for the change you want for you!

Here are three areas of work that can help you live into this prayer when you are ready:

1) Wisdom

- **Discern what you can and cannot control.**

  - Pause or stop.

  - Ground self in the present moment.

  - Connect with your diaphragmatic breath.

  - Allow your improved calmness to help you think more clearly, completely, and realistically.

  - Now ask your self: *What in this situation with this person can I control?*

  - Now ask your self: *What in this situation with this person is not in my control?*

2) Serenity

- **Act on what you can control.**

  - Notice what you need, want, feel, and believe. To help with this:

    » Think about the scale you studied in **Handout 6: Self/Other Balance Scale**.

    » Consider the line down the page activity you learned about in **Client Worksheet 14: Separating Me from You**.

  - Then, with clarity from discerning what you can control and your increased awareness of what is yours, act on your own behalf to cultivate *your* life.

3) Courage

- **Let go of what you cannot control.**

  - Increase your awareness of when you are dealing with something beyond your control. Your internal cues—or the considerations from the previous bullet—can help you know when you need to let go. So can the balance scale and the line down the page activity.

  - Absorb the limitations of what you can do for or with someone else.

  - Grieve the reality of these limitations. This reality will free you, though it may sadden or frustrate you at first. **Handout 13: Skills for Grieving** can help you with this process.

  - Cultivate a personal way or spiritual belief system so you can release what you cannot control. Review the ideas you created for ways you can let go in **Client Worksheet 16: Releasing**.

  - Think of something that is not in your control that you are ready to release. Use idea(s) from **worksheet 16** to help you courageously let go of whatever you have discerned is not yours to control.

Strategy 62

Foster a secure attachment with self.

Everything in this chapter on self-attunement is designed to help your clients establish a secure attachment with self. This final strategy pulls together all the other self-attunement strategies with the hopeful message that we truly can have a relationship with our self that offers a reliable source of safety, attunement, and responsiveness.

This secure attachment with self does not discount the possibility of having such a relationship with others, but it is foundational to an individual's mental health to know that *they* will always be there for self. A secure attachment with self creates the possibility of healthier relationships with others, relationships where the codependent does not need to compulsively fix, please, or control. Instead, the codependent in self-recovery can interact in an adult-to-adult way, fully connected with self as they listen and respond to, love and live with others.

The following **Self-Attunement Exercises 4–5: Establishing a Secure Attachment with Self** will integrate self-attunement exercises 1–3 with two additional exercises, and it can help your client deepen and solidify their ongoing relationship-with-self.

Establishing a Secure Attachment with Self

This exercise pulls together the things you have been learning about self-attunement to establish a secure attachment with self, which is essential to your relationship-with-self. Use these exercises in the order they're listed, as they build upon each other. Daily practices like these are important for change.

To start, review the exercises that you've already learned and practiced:

- **Self-Attunement Exercise 1: Fostering Your Internal Connections through Conscious Awareness**
- **Self-Attunement Exercise 2: Meet, Greet, and Respond to Your Gatekeepers**
- **Self-Attunement Exercise 3: Fostering Your Supportive Self-Regard**

Then add the following new exercises:

SELF-ATTUNEMENT EXERCISE 4
Consistently Show Up for You

The greater goal of this self-attunement work is to be in connection with your self in ongoing ways, not just occasionally or when you are distressed or pressed. If we only seek out a friend when we need something from them, the relationship can sour. In contrast, consistent and ongoing connection supports secure relationship growth. Consistency teaches us that we can count on something. We want to count on our self to be there for our self.

Practice: *Over the course of a day, see how many times you are able to pause and connect with self in an interested, caring way: How am I? What do I need? How can I reasonably give that to my self?*

SELF-ATTUNEMENT EXERCISE 5
Anchor in Self

Self-recovery offers a safe haven within you for experiencing both the storms and delights of life, a place to go to for compassion, calm presence, confidence, and care. Anchoring in self means developing a clear understanding and commitment to self–body, mind, emotions, and spirit—and staying connected with these aspects of self through attentive, supportive, and responsive behaviors as you live with and love others.

Practice: *Let's learn to anchor in self using the following meditation:*

An anchor holds a boat in place. The boat may rock or move around a bit, depending on the length of the rope to which it is attached. Nevertheless, the boat stays within the range of its anchoring, sometimes being pulled to the far edges of that range but not beyond. If we happen to be on that boat, we trust that the anchor will keep us safe and where we want to be.

Similarly, anchoring in self is not rigid; as with the boat's anchor, there is some range in where you are anchored. This range allows you to hear the other person, consider what they are saying, and remember the relationship you have and want to have with them. But listening does not mean pulling up your anchor and drifting away with the other person, leaving your relationship-with-self behind. Anchoring in self means knowing that you can stay within your internal safe haven and enjoy its secure benefits as you meet life's challenges and opportunities (Johnston, 2020).

Cynthia and Her Relationship-with-Self

When I introduced this idea of a relationship-with-self to Cynthia, she was unfamiliar with it; she even thought it was weird. She chuckled somewhat uncomfortably. I explained that we work hard to have relationships with others, sometimes so hard that we leave our self behind. Then I suggested, "What if we also had a relationship-with-self that we considered as well?"

Cynthia asked, "How would that help me with my codependency?"

I answered, "Having a relationship-with-self is the heart of our recovery from codependency. It means caring enough about our self that we actively factor our self into the relationships and activities in our daily life."

Cynthia was willing to work with the five self-attunement exercises. Even though she found it difficult to use them outside of session, she was grateful for the relief and clarity they gave her in our sessions. Those experiences were enough to keep her working on her relationship-with-self.

1. ***Foster your internal connection:*** *Cynthia did not immediately take to pausing and connecting with self. A busy woman, she always had a full to-do list, and stopping was not on that list. But she was interested in being in better balance with her daughter, so she practiced internal connecting twice each day for three to five minutes. She improved her ability to quiet her thoughts and check in with her four areas of self. This gave her a fuller awareness and understanding of self and helped her to see more options for responding to her daughter and self.*

2. ***Meet, greet, and respond to your gatekeepers:*** *Cynthia definitely ran into her gatekeepers, and she became quite interested in them. In the past, she always let the gatekeepers deny her access to self or chase her away. Shame and guilt were common gatekeepers for her. Worry and fear were regulars as well. Cynthia learned to notice, name, and converse with the gatekeepers who appeared. She even chose to give some of them personal names. As a result of this relationship-building with her gatekeepers, Cynthia was able to access her self more often and comfortably.*

3. ***Foster your supportive self-regard:*** *"Supportive" became an important word for Cynthia in terms of self-regard. She was surprised at how undermining her usual thoughts were: "You will say it wrong." "You are not doing enough." "You are a bad mother." Through conscious awareness and with honesty, Cynthia modified her self-talk: "I know what I am saying, and I believe it." "I am doing plenty." "I am a good mother." As Cynthia's relationship-with-self grew, these supportive self-statements became more natural and true for her.*

4. ***Consistently show up for you:*** *Cynthia saw how consistently she showed up for her daughter. She would have her phone with her all the time, immediately respond to texts, and drop everything for Jenna. She realized she was not doing anything to this extent for herself. To change this, she set an alarm on her phone every four hours to re-mind her to stop, check in with her self, and see if she could do anything to make her life better in that moment. Cynthia*

said that this connection with self could change her day and her mood, making it easier for her to go for a walk or make plans with a friend. Over time, her consistent check-ins with self became a new pattern that reinforced Cynthia's belief that she can count on Cynthia.

- **Anchor in self:** *Cynthia liked the notion of anchoring in self. She occasionally experienced the security and safety it offers. But she remained subject to the storms of her daughter's life, and sometimes her self-anchor pulled up in middle of those storms. I offered patience and compassion as we worked on these challenges. I helped her to understand that progress is often two steps forward, one step back. Change is difficult and possible with consistent and committed practice of these exercises.*

Insights and Intentions

Consider the strategies introduced in this chapter:

54. Understand **self-attunement**.

55. Identify **desired qualities** of a relationship-with-self.

56. Learn to **access** self.

57. Sustain a healthy **internal focus**.

58. Meet their **gatekeepers**.

59. Cultivate **paths** to their relationship-with-self.

60. Establish supportive **self-regard**.

61. Act on things in **their control**.

62. Foster a **secure attachment with self**.

What have you learned in this chapter about helping your clients develop self-attunement *with care?*

_____

_____

Which handouts or exercises in this chapter seem particularly useful in your work with codependent clients?

_____

_____

Have you had any realizations about your self?

_____

_____

Are there worksheets or exercises in this chapter you might intentionally bring to your practice or apply in your own life?

_____

_____

Part IV

Self-Recovery as a Way of Being

You have carefully studied and worked with the four elements of self-recovery: understanding, awareness, competence, and attunement. Each element is full of skills and insights that can help your codependent client keep their focus on self in new and effective ways. Nevertheless, they are likely still challenged by the draw of the external—the needs, requests, worries, and upsets of others. This is normal for someone who is changing long-standing patterns of thoughts and actions. Your task is to help them take the next, most profound step: making self-recovery their way of being.

"Way of being" means they are connected with self on an ongoing basis. It means they more naturally stop and consider self. They actively employ guilt management skills and assertiveness as they move through their days. They intentionally deliver supportive self-statements. Their connections with self are not visits; they are able to live in their garden of self. They have come to know their gatekeepers and have workable, even supportive, relationships with them. They know how to meet and greet a new gatekeeper who may not have shown up before. They value their evolving relationship-with-self and find that it gives them strength and security.

CHAPTER 10

Strategies to Help the Codependent Client Sustain Their Self-Recovery

Many of us know the experience of learning something we think is a great idea but then never revisiting that idea again. It remains theoretical, not practical, and it certainly does not become our way of being. The essential ingredients of change—awareness, willingness, and intentionality—apply in helping your client move toward self-recovery as their way of being. All three ingredients are needed, but intentionality carries the weight of moving forward.

Intentionality means creating the time and energy for the practice required. It involves commitment to self and to this process, which rewires your client's long-lost or self-denied internal focus. This chapter offers four strategies to help your client move toward making self-recovery their new and improved way of being. The four strategies are briefly described in the following paragraphs. Then, integrate each of the strategies using **Client Worksheet 18: Self-Recovery as *Your* Way of Being**—a four-part worksheet with specific exercises and journaling for each strategy.

Strategy 63

Maintain **conscious connections** with self-recovery.

Self-recovery work invites your client to be in conscious contact with their therapy goals, the four elements of self-recovery, and their gatekeepers. Staying in contact with these foundational pieces of self-recovery provides a basic map that will help them make and sustain the changes they desire in their intra- or interpersonal patterns.

Keeping their goals in mind will help your client stay on their new course. They will also benefit from remembering the four elements of self-recovery and each element's associated strategies that support their goals. And, of course, they will have ongoing interactions with their gatekeepers as they access self. Helping them become increasingly familiar with these various parts of self will help your client develop a more cooperative internal community, which in turn offers greater peace and efficacy to their relationship-with-self.

Client Worksheet 18, Part 1: Conscious Connections with My Self-Recovery, can help your client plan their conscious connections with their goals, the four elements of self-recovery, and their gatekeepers.

Strategy 64

Practice **internal focus** daily.

Making the shift from a dominantly other-centered way of being to compassionately considering self along with others requires regular practice. Regular practice requires belief in the importance of this change and commitment to the strategies and exercises that foster balance with self and others. As your client establishes daily practices to pause, connect, and notice self, make sure they see the value and commitment this takes. They may well have gatekeepers who are restless and doubtful that these practices will help. Spending time with those gatekeepers to work through such differences will help your clients make good use of their daily practices. Over time, their daily practices can evolve into self-recovery as a way of being.

Client Worksheet 18, Part 2: Daily Practices to Develop My Internal Focus offers your client a reminder list of practices to cultivate their internal focus. There is also space for them to design other practices that work for them.

Strategy 65

Develop **ongoing ways** to use internal focus.

What does the shift from "daily practice" to "way of being" look like? It looks like your client tuning into self in a number of ways over the course of the day, naturally and spontaneously. Your client notices self amid their daily activities. When they have a strong emotion, they pause and connect with self. If they are confused, they settle into self. This shift indicates that they have developed regular self-attunement that supports them, that they trust, and that feels good and reliable.

Here are two ongoing ways for your client to use their internal focus:

- **Notice self in the moment:** Invite your client to notice self in both quiet and active moments. In quiet moments, their noticing can be a caring curiosity, perhaps a moment for supportive self-regard. In active moments, when either an external or internal stimulus has drawn their energy and focus away from self, invite them to pause and reconnect with self. Help them create a space between the stimulus and their reactions by reconnecting with their reasons, values, goals, and relationship-with-self. This gives them the opportunity to respond rather than react and to make their desired changes on their own behalf.

- **Intervene on your own behalf:** As you know, an intervention is a caring process intended to connect a loved one with the addiction treatment they need. It's rare for an intervention to be arranged for a codependent person . . . but sometimes we need one! Self-recovery gives us the knowledge, skills, and opportunities to intervene on our own behalf when we have gone too far, we have lost our self, or we are not well. Once we notice self, we can act in ways that support our self-recovery: we can stop, leave, take a break, say something different, or say less. When we are with our self, not beside our self, we can choose to do something different for our own good in that moment when change and growth are possible. Intervening on our own behalf is how we recover our self.

Client Worksheet 18, Part 3: Ongoing Ways to Use My Internal Focus guides your client through these two specific ways of making internal focus their way of being.

Strategy 66

Foster their relationship-with-self.

"Foster" is such a lovely word. It is gentle and loving. It feels supportive and encouraging. It implies growth. We foster children, animals, and organizations. Why not foster our self, too? **Client Worksheet 18, Part 4: Practices to Develop My Relationship-with-Self** offers several ideas to encourage this fostering of self.

To start, invite your client to assess their progress. Over the course of sessions, it is possible to lose track of the good work being accomplished. Join them in intentionally looking at their original goals, encourage them to notice what is better for them, and help them absorb what is working and the changes they are experiencing. I promise they will find improvements, and this attending-to-self supports long-term recovery.

Creating self-statements that accurately reflect their growth is also a good way to foster relationship-with-self. These self-statements can come from their assessed progress, or they can be prompted by completing sentences like, "I used to _____, but now I _____." "I am noticing I _____." "What is working for me is _____."

Re-mind your client that noting their progress *is* self-awareness; absorbing it and believing in self *is* self-attunement. These actions foster their relationship-with-self until ultimately, they will do this self-work on their own. They will naturally connect with, offer support to, and respond reliably to self. They will know their path. They will have their skills. Their relationship-with-self will be comfortable and secure.

My Plan: Practices that Support Self-Recovery as a Way of Being

Congratulations on all the work you have been doing on your own behalf! Codependency can make us so focused on our relationship with someone else that we may walk away from our relationship-with-self. Learning to stay connected with your self and respond with patience and kindness is the heart of self-recovery.

Through this workbook you have used a number of handouts, worksheets, and exercises to learn new things and to practice new ways of thinking, handling your emotions, expressing your self, and acting on what is true for you. Great work!

Now you are invited to identify practices that will help you continue this work and make self-recovery your way of being. This means you will actively pause, connect with self, discern, and respond until it all becomes second nature for you. You know that being balanced in your care of self and others can improve your mood, outlook, and relationships, and you are committed to living in this way. You are anchored in the safe, secure haven of self and know how to return to it as life's storms pull you out to sea.

What follows is an opportunity to create a plan for solidifying your self-recovery work. The four parts of your plan involve information and practices that will help your self-recovery become an increasingly natural and satisfying way of being for you.

Part 1: Conscious Connections with My Self-Recovery

My Goals

What are your goals for your self? Being clear about your goals and keeping them in mind helps to keep you on your desired course.

_____

_____

_____

_____

The Four Elements of Self-Recovery

The self-recovery image reminds you of the four elements involved in self-recovery. Remember, these elements are not a list where you complete one element and move on to the next. Rather, you will use these four elements as needed—situation by situation. Sometimes you will need to increase your self-awareness, while other times you will use a new skill you learned in self-competence. You will always be gaining self-understanding and expanding the ways you self-attune. Your self-recovery process is active and ongoing. This is how you make progress and strengthen your new internal and external patterns.

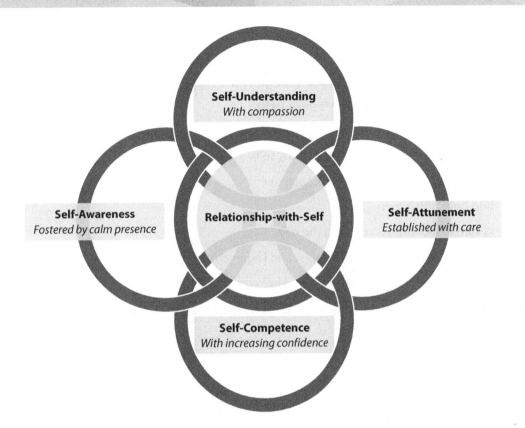

Self-Understanding
With compassion

Self-Awareness
Fostered by calm presence

Relationship-with-Self

Self-Attunement
Established with care

Self-Competence
With increasing confidence

What is one strategy from each of these four elements of self-recovery you can use to support your goals?

- **Self-understanding:** _____

  _____

- **Self-awareness:** _____

  _____

- **Self-competence:** _____

  _____

- **Self-attunement:** _____

  _____

My Gatekeepers

When you feel discouraged or stuck, go within and meet the gatekeepers who may be there protecting you. Use the ideas you have been taught to see if the two of you can work out a trusting agreement that allows you to move forward with your life. What is your experience with your gatekeepers? Has anything changed in your relationship with your gatekeepers?

_____

_____

My Homework

Self-assignments are a good way to deepen and solidify your work. Here are some homework ideas with spaces for you to create your own self-recovery assignments. Place a check mark by the ones that interest you. Then circle the ones you will do on a regular basis.

- ☐ Journaling whatever I want
- ☐ Drawing, coloring, or painting to express my self
- ☐ Finding and reading a book that might help me
- ☐ Spending time with a friend
- ☐ Making sure to move around during the day
- ☐ Working on one assignment my therapist and I agreed on
- ☐ Researching something I may be interested in
- ☐ Checking out something I have been curious about, like a park, restaurant, store, or new walking path.
- ☐ _____
- ☐ _____

Part 2: Daily Practices to Develop My Internal Focus

You have learned to shift your awareness to your body, mind, emotions, and spirit. This is the essential foundation for codependency recovery. You have practiced exercises that restore you to the present moment and studied ways to access self. Daily practices can help you make this shift to within a more natural part of you.

Daily Practices

Here are some daily practice ideas for you to add your own plans. Place a check mark by the ones that appeal to you. Then circle the ones you will do on a regular basis.

- ☐ Reading daily reflections that re-mind and support my changes
- ☐ Actively journaling (whatever that means to me)
- ☐ Intentionally pausing and connecting with self, checking in on all four areas of self
- ☐ Intentionally coming to the present through mindful breathing, grounding practices, or my senses
- ☐ Connecting with people who understand the work I am doing on my own behalf
- ☐ Connecting with my strengths, adult parts, and wise self
- ☐ Connecting with my gratitude
- ☐ Connecting with me and responding to what I need in that moment, if possible
- ☐ _____
- ☐ _____
- ☐ _____

Part 3: Ongoing Ways to Use My Internal Focus

As you get more familiar and comfortable with connecting with you, you are invited to have an ongoing, organic connection with your self throughout your day, without having to stop and intentionally practice.

Ongoing Practices

- **Notice self in the moment:** Whatever has drawn your energy and focus—whether internal or external stimuli—make sure to check in with self in that present moment. Your reactions to stimuli that disconnect you from your self are solid cues to turn, go within, and safely and calmly reconnect with self.

  Can you imagine noticing self in the moment on and off throughout your day? What cues—thoughts, feelings, body sensations—might direct you to go within and anchor there?

  _____

  _____

- **Intervene on your own behalf:** Do something to take care of you in the moment when you notice you are losing your self. Stop. Leave. Take a break. Say something different. Say less. Act in a way that supports your health and self-recovery.

  What do you think of this idea to intervene on your own behalf?

  _____

  _____

  When might it be good to intervene on your own behalf? What would you do in that moment?

  _____

  _____

Part 4: Practices to Develop My Relationship-with-Self

Noticing what you are accomplishing is very important. Recognizing your progress and really taking it in supports long-term change. Noting your progress _is_ self-awareness. Absorbing it and believing in you _is_ self-attunement. Your secure relationship-with-self grows from these actions.

Self-Assessment

To see your progress, look back at **Handout 7: Assessing for Overfunctioning for Others/Underfunctioning for Self**. Answer them again, with your current understanding of your relationship-with-self. Do you notice any changes in you?

_____

_____

Self-Statements

Here are some self-statements to help you stay in touch with you, your goals, and your growth. Feel free to add some of your own statements, too.

- I used to _____, but now I _____.

- I am noticing that I now _____.

- What is working for me is _____.

- I feel good when I am able to _____.

- I surprise myself when I _____.

- _____

- _____

- _____

My Relationship-with-Self

Create reminders of your relationship with you. Have active, ongoing self-connectivity with curiosity and willingness, trust and consistency, playfulness and fun.

How will you stay in touch with your relationship with you? What will help you to remember and sustain this most important relationship—your relationship with your self?

_____

_____

Insights and Intentions

Consider the strategies introduced in this chapter:

63. Maintain **conscious connections** with self-recovery.

64. Practice **internal focus** daily.

65. Develop **ongoing ways** to use internal focus.

66. **Foster** their relationship-with-self.

What have you learned in this chapter about helping your clients sustain their self-recovery?

_____

_____

_____

Which strategies or exercises in this chapter seem particularly useful in your work with codependent clients?

_____

_____

_____

Have you had any realizations about your self?

_____

_____

_____

Are there strategies or exercises in this chapter you might intentionally bring to your practice or apply in your own life?

_____

_____

_____

Resources

For your convenience, purchasers can download and print the worksheets from **pesipubs.com/codepwkbk**

Al-Anon Family Groups. (1987). *One day at a time in Al-Anon.*

Bermúdez, J. A., Garcia, L. H., & Castillo, M. M. A. (2017) The level of well-being in families attending al-anon groups and its effect on the attention of their alcohol dependent relatives. *MOJ Addiction Medicine & Therapy, 4*(1). https://doi.org/10.15406/mojamt.2017.04.00067

Artemtseva, N. G., & Malkina, M. A. (2022). Cognitive mistakes of codependents as a way to protect against uncertainty. *Vestnik of Samara State Technical University Psychological and Pedagogical Sciences, 19*(1), 153–166. https://doi.org/10.17673/vsgtu-pps.2022.1.11

Bacon, I., Reynolds, F., McKay, E., & McIntyre, A. (2017). 'The Lady of Shalott': Insights gained from using visual methods and interviews exploring the lived experience of codependency. *Qualitative Methods in Psychology Bulletin, 23.* https://doi.org/ 10.53841/bpsqmip.2017.1.23.24

Baranowsky, A. B., & Gentry, J. E. (2023). *Trauma practice: A cognitive behavioral somatic therapy* (4th ed.). Hogrefe Publishing.

Bartholomew, K., & Horowitz, L. M. (1991). Attachment styles among young adults: A test of a four-category model. *Journal of Personality and Social Psychology, 61*(2), 226–244. https://doi.org/10.1037//0022-3514.61.2.226

Beattie, M. (1990). *The language of letting go: Daily meditations for codependents.* Harper & Row.

Bray, J. H., Williamson, D. S. & Malone, P. E. (1984). Personal authority in the family system: Development of a questionnaire to measure personal authority in intergenerational family processes. *Journal of Marital and Family Therapy, 10*(2), 167–178. https://doi.org/10.1111/j.1752-0606.1984.tb00007.x

Brown, B. (2006). Shame resilience theory: A grounded theory study on women and shame. *Families in Society, 87*(1), 43–52. https://doi.org/10.1606/1044-3894.3483

Central Recovery. (2017). *Discover recovery: A comprehensive addiction recovery workbook.*

Child & Adolescent Health Measurement Initiative. (n.d.). *ACEs resource packet: Adverse childhood experiences (ACEs) basics.* https://www.childhealthdata.org/docs/default-source/cahmi/aces-resource-packet_all-pages_12_06-16112336f3c0266255aab2ff00001023b1.pdf

Fuller, J. A., & Warner, R. M. (2000). Family stressors as predictors of codependency. *Genetic, Social, and General Psychology Monographs, 126*(1), 5–22.

Graham, L. (2018). *Resilience: Powerful practices for bouncing back from disappointment, difficulty, and even disaster.* New World Library.

Happ, Z., Bodó-Varga, Z, Bandi, S. A., Kiss, E. C., Nagy, L., & Csókási, K. (2023). How codependency affects dyadic coping, relationship perception and life satisfaction. *Current Psychology, 42,* 15688–15695. https://doi.org/10.1007/s12144-022-02875-9

Hazan, C., & Shaver, P. (1987). Romantic love conceptualized as an attachment process. *Journal of Personality and Social Psychology, 52*(3), 511–524. https://doi.org/10.1037//0022-3514.52.3.511

Johnston, N. L. (2012). *My life as a border collie: Freedom from codependency.* Central Recovery Press.

Lampis, J., Cataudella, S., Busonera, A., & Skowron, E. A. (2017). The role of differentiation of self and dyadic adjustment in predicting codependency. *Contemporary Family Therapy, 39*(1), 62–72. https://doi.org/10.1007/s10591-017-9403-4

Nhất Hạnh, T. (2011). *Peace is every breath: A practice for our busy lives.* HarperOne.

Rotter, J. B. (1954). *Social learning and clinical psychology.* Prentice-Hall. https://doi.org/10.1037/10788-000

Tranberg, M., Andersson, M., Nilbert, M., & Rasmussen, B. H. (2019). Co-afflicted but invisible: A qualitative study of perceptions among informal caregivers in cancer care. *Journal of Health Psychology, 26*(11). https://doi.org/10.1177/1359105319890407

Yoder, B. (1990). *The Recovery Resource Book.* Simon & Schuster.

Zielinski, M., D'Aniello, C., Bradshaw, S. D., Shumway, S. T., & Edwards, L. (2022). Differentiation of self in family members' of SUD loved ones: An analysis of prefrontal cortex activation. *Contemporary Family Therapy, 44*(3), 250–266. https://doi.org/10.1007/s10591-022-09639-4

References

Ainsworth, M. D. S., & Bell, S. M. (1970). Attachment, exploration, and separation: Illustrated by the behavior of one-year-olds in a strange situation. *Child Development, 41*(1), 49–67. https://doi.org/10.2307/1127388

Ainsworth, M. D. S., Blebar, M. C., Waters, E., & Wall., S. (2015). *Patterns of attachment: A psychological study of the strange situation.* Psychology Press. (Original work published 1979).

American Psychiatric Association. (2013). *Diagnostic and statistical manual of mental disorders* (5th ed.). https://doi.org/10.1176/appi.books.9780890425596

Anderson, F. (2023). To forgive or not to forgive. [Digital seminar]. *Psychotherapy Networker Symposium.* https://catalog.psychotherapynetworker.org/item/to-forgive-forgive-releasing-pain-relational-trauma-120438

Bacon, I., McKay, E., Reynolds, F., & McIntyre, A. (2020a). The lived experience of codependency: An interpretative phenomenological analysis. *International Journal of Mental Health and Addiction, 18*(3), 754–771. https://doi.org/10.1007/s11469-018-9983-8

Bacon, I., McKay, E., Reynolds, F., & McIntyre, A. (2020b). An examination of the lived experience of attending twelve-step groups for co-dependency. *International Journal of Mental Health and Addiction, 19*(5), 1646–1661. https://doi.org/10.1007/s11469-020-00253-9

Bacon, I., & Conway, J. (2023). Co-dependency and enmeshment—a fusion of concepts. *International Journal of Mental Health and Addiction, 21*, 3594–3603. https://doi.org/10.1007/s11469-022-00810-4

Beattie, M. (1987). *Codependent no more: How to stop controlling others and start caring for yourself.* Hazelden.

Beck, J. S. (2021). *Cognitive behavior therapy: Basics and beyond* (3rd ed.). The Guilford Press.

Black, C. (2020). *It will never happen to me* (3rd ed.). Central Recovery Press. (Original work published 1981).

Bowlby, J. (1988). *A secure base: Parent-child attachment and healthy human development.* Routledge.

Bowen, M. (1978). *Family therapy in clinical practice.* Jason Aronson.

Brown, B. (2007). *I thought it was just me (but it isn't): Telling the truth about perfectionism, inadequacy, and power.* Gotham Books.

Brown, B. (2018). *Dare to lead: Brave work. Tough conversations. Whole hearts.* Vermilion.

Burns, D. D. (2020). *Feeling great: The revolutionary new treatment for depression and anxiety.* PESI Publishing.

Cermak, T. L. (1986). *Diagnosing and treating co-dependence: A guide for professionals who work with chemical dependents, their spouses and children.* Johnson Institute Books.

Co-Dependents Anonymous. (2011). *Patterns and characteristics of codependence.* http://coda.org/index.cfm/meeting-materials1/patterns-andcharacteristics-2011

Dana, D. (2018). *The polyvagal theory in therapy: Engaging the rhythm of regulation.* W. W. Norton.

Dana, D. (2020). *Polyvagal exercises for safety and connection: 50 client-centered practices.* W. W. Norton.

Dear, G. E., Roberts, C. M., & Lange, L. (2004). Defining codependency: An analysis of published definitions. In S. Shohov (Ed.), *Advances in psychology research, 34,* 189–205. Nova Science Publishers.

Dear, G. E., & Roberts, C. M. (2005). Validation of the Holyoake codependency index. *The Journal of Psychology, 139*(4), 293–313. https://doi.org/10.3200/JRLP.139.4.293-314

Fagan-Pryor, E. C., & Haber, L C. (1992). Codependency: Another name for Bowen's undifferentiated self. *Perspectives in Psychiatric Care, 28*(4), 24–28. https://doi.org/10.1111/j.1744-6163.1992.tb00389.x

Felitti, V. J., Anda, R. F., Nordenberg, D., Williamson, D. F., Spitz, A. M., Edwards, V., Koss, M. P., & Marks, J. S. (1998). Relationship of childhood abuse and household dysfunction to many of the leading causes of death in adults: The Adverse Childhood Experiences (ACE) Study. *American Journal of Preventive Medicine, 14*(4), 245–258. https://doi.org/10.1016/S0749-3797(98)00017-8

Fischer, J. L., Spann, L., & Crawford, D. (1991). Measuring codependency. *Alcoholism Treatment Quarterly, 8*(1), 87–100. https://doi.org/10.1300/J020V08N01_06

Fisher, G. L., & Harrison, T. C. (2018). *Substance abuse: Information for school counselors, social workers, therapists, and counselors* (6th ed.). Pearson.

Fisher, J. (2021). *Transforming the living legacy of trauma: A workbook for survivors and therapists.* PESI Publishing.

Fisher, J. (2022). *The living legacy of trauma flip chart: A psychoeducational in-session tool for clients and therapists.* PESI Publishing.

Gentry, J. E. (2021). Trauma recovery scale. *Upstream Counseling.* https://upstreamcounseling.org/wp-content/uploads/2021/05/BLANK-TRS.pdf.

Gilbert, R. M. (2004). *The eight concepts of Bowen theory: A new way of thinking about the individual and the group.* Leading Systems Press.

Greenberg, M. (2016). *The stress-proof brain: Master your emotional response to stress using mindfulness and neuroplasticity.* New Harbinger.

Hanson, R. (n.d.). *How to take in the good.* https://www.rickhanson.net/how-to-take-in-the-good/?cn-reloaded=1

Hanson, R. (2009). *Buddha's brain: The practical science of happiness, love, and wisdom.* New Harbinger.

Hanson, R. (2013). *Hardwiring happiness: The new brain science of contentment, calm, and confidence.* Harmony.

Hölzel, B. K., Carmody, J., Vangel, M., Congleton, C., Yerramsetti, S. M., Gard, T., & Lazar, S. W. (2011). Mindfulness practice leads to increases in regional brain gray matter density. *Psychiatry Research, 191*(1), 36–43. https://doi.org/10.1016/j.pscychresns.2010.08.006

Johnston, N. L. (2020). *Disentangle: When you've lost your self in someone else* (2nd ed.). Central Recovery Press. (Original work published 2011).

Kabat-Zinn, J. (2013). *Full catastrophe living* (Rev. ed.). Bantam Books. (Original work published 1990).

Kerr, M. E. (2019). *One family's story: A primer on Bowen theory.* The Bowen Center for the Study of the Family.

Kessler, D. (2019). *Finding meaning: The sixth stage of grief.* Scribner.

Kübler-Ross, E. (1969). *On death and dying.* Macmillan.

Lampis, J. & Cataudella, S. (2019). Adult attachment and differentiation of self-constructs: A possible dialogue? *Contemporary Family Therapy, 41*(3), 227–235. https://doi.org/10.1007/s10591-019-09489-7

Main, M., & Solomon, J. (1986). Discovery of an insecure-disorganized/disoriented attachment pattern. In T. B. Brazelton & M. W. Yogman (Eds.), *Affective Development in Infancy* (pp. 95–124). Ablex Publishing.

Marks, A. D. G., Blore, R. L., Hine, D. W., & Dear, G. E. (2012). Development and validation of a revised measure of codependency. *Australian Journal of Psychology, 64*(3), 119–127. https://doi.org/10.1111/j.1742-9536.2011.00034.x

Maslow, A. H. (1943). A theory of human motivation. *Psychological Review, 50*(4), 370–396. https://doi.org/10.1037/h0054346

Mellody, P. (2003). *Facing codependence: What it is, where it comes from, how it sabotages our lives.* HarperOne. (Original work published 1989).

Miller, A. (1981). *The drama of the gifted child: The search for the true self.* Basic Books.

Morrow, K., & Spencer, E. D. (2018). *CBT for anxiety: A step-by-step training manual for the treatment of fear, panic, worry and OCD.* PESI Publishing.

National Council of Juvenile and Family Court Judges. (2006). *Finding your ACE score.* https://www.ncjfcj.org/wp-content/uploads/2006/10/Finding-Your-Ace-Score.pdf.

Nhất Hạnh, T. (1991). *Peace is every step: The path of mindfulness in everyday life.* Bantam Books.

Norwood, R. (2008). *Women who love too much: When you keep wishing and hoping he'll change.* Pocket Books. (Original work published 1985).

Porges, S. (2011). *The Polyvagal theory: Neurophysiological foundations of emotions, attachment, communication, and self-regulation.* W. W. Norton.

Prochaska, J., & DiClemente, C. C. (1983). Stages and processes of self-change in smoking: Toward an integrative model of change. *Journal of Consulting and Clinical Psychology, 51*(3), 390–395. https://doi.org/10.1037//0022-006x.51.3.390

Real, T. (2022). *What is RLT?* [Video]. Relational Life Institute. https://relationallife.com/level-1-training-what-is-rlt/?utm_source=ontraport&utm_medium=email&utm_campaign=level1email3

Schwartz, A. (2016). *The complex PTSD workbook: A mind-body approach to regaining emotional control and becoming whole.* Althea Press.

Schwartz, A. (2021). *The complex PTSD treatment manual: An integrative, mind-body approach to trauma recovery.* PESI Publishing.

Schwartz, R. C., & Sweezy, M. (2020). *Internal family systems therapy* (2nd ed.). The Guilford Press.

Sweeton, J. (2019). *Trauma treatment toolbox: 165 brain-changing tips, tools & handouts to move therapy forward.* PESI Publishing.

Tawwab, N. G. (2023). *How boundaries can save your family relationships.* [Digital seminar]. Psychotherapy Networker Symposium. https://catalog.psychotherapynetworker.org/item/how-boundaries-save-family-relationships-120434

van der Kolk, B. (2014). *The body keeps the score: Brain, mind, and body in the healing of trauma.* Penguin Books.

Walker, P. (2013). *Complex PTSD: From surviving to thriving: A guide and map for recovering from childhood trauma.* CreateSpace Independent Publishing Platform.

Wegscheider-Cruse, S. (1989). *Another chance: Hope and health for the alcoholic family* (2nd ed.). Science & Behavior Books.

Woititz, J. G. (1990). *Adult children of alcoholics, expanded edition.* Health Communications.

Zelvin, E., (2004). Treating the partners of substance abusers. In S. L. A. Straussner (Ed.), *Clinical work with substance abusing clients* (pp. 264–283). The Guilford Press.

Acknowledgments

This workbook is the product of 35 years of personal and professional work. Its creation is a story of ever-evolving projects and writings based out of a rural community in Virginia—now offered to the larger world. Many people and opportunities along the way have made the development of this important workbook on codependency possible, and to each of them, I give my heartfelt thanks:

- Clarisse Harrison and Martha Brinson, my high school humanities teachers who helped me get started as a writer, as painful as it was at times with me crying in the supply closet as Miss Harrison tried to help me understand her critiques of my writing.

- Nadia Kuley, who in 1988 recognized my talents as a therapist and offered me clinical opportunities to grow and shine in my work.

- Mentors and friends over three decades who have helped me understand codependency from the inside out: Toby, Ruth, Lois, Cindy, Molly, Margaret, Sally, Dave, Dan, and Linda. Through many a conversation, walks and talks, and weekend getaways, I learned how to find and live in serenity more often than not.

- Every client, workshop participant, and conference session attendee who shared their stories and questions with me as they learned how to kindly consider and respond to self.

- Margaret Cress, for two decades of delightful work together designing and facilitating our Codependence Camp and all the campers who have brought curiosity, willingness, and laughter to camp and their own growth over these years.

- The Virginia Counselors Association and the Virginia Summer Institute for Addiction Studies, for the many opportunities to present at their conferences, which inspired me to further develop and clarify my clinical work with codependency in order to teach others.

- Nancy Schenck and Valerie Killeen at Central Recovery Press, who in 2010 recognized the value of my work on codependency and published two of my books on this topic.

- Zachary Taylor, Kate Sample, Ryan Bartholomew, Josh Becker, Chelsea Thompson, Alissa Schneider, G. Panzer, and Emily Dyer at PESI, who have been enthusiastically cheering me on since 2019 to create this workbook. Their interest in codependency, amazing abilities to synthesize and edit my material, and constant respect and kindness all made this project a gift of a lifetime for me.

- Loving thanks to my daughter and her partner for providing listening ears, supportive questions, and their back porch in Boston, which served as my morning writer's retreat during some of the early phases of this workbook's creation.

- Finally, special thanks to my husband of 42 years for patiently listening to me as I lived through the joys and challenges of this project. Thank you for our nightly dinners and conversations and for always giving me space to create and find my own way.

About the Author

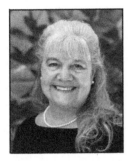 **Nancy L. Johnston, MS, LPC, LSATP, MAC, NCC**, is a licensed professional counselor and licensed substance abuse treatment practitioner in private practice in Lexington, VA. With 46 years of clinical experience, Nancy is a master addiction counselor and an American Mental Health Counselors Association (AMHCA) diplomate in substance abuse and co-occurring disorders.

She has authored two books on codependency published by Central Recovery Press: *Disentangle: When You've Lost Your Self in Someone Else,* 2nd Edition (2020) and *My Life as a Border Collie: Freedom from Codependency* (2012).

In addition to this workbook, Nancy has two digital seminars produced with PESI for clinicians on treating codependency: "Codependence: Treatment Strategies for Clients Who Lose Themselves in Others" (2020) and "The Codependency Treatment Guide: CBT, Somatic Strategies and More to Disentangle Clients from Dysfunctional Relationships and Recover Self" (2022).

Nancy remains active in her counseling practice, working with individuals, couples, and families. She offers online self-recovery workshops and delights in designing and facilitating Codependence Camp twice a year at a retreat site in Virginia. Codependence Camp has been in operation since 2004.

Over the past 20 years, Nancy has presented at numerous conferences including the Cape Cod Symposium on Addictive Disorders, the Carolinas Conference for Addiction and Recovery, Addiction: Focus on Women, the Virginia Summer Institute for Addiction Studies, the American Mental Health Counselors Association's Annual Conference, the Virginia Counselors Association's Annual Conference, and Specialty Docket Training for the Virginia Supreme Court.

Nancy writes from her country home on a river in the Valley of Virginia. When she is not working with clients, writing, or teaching, Nancy enjoys extended time with family and friends, gardening, writing haiku, traveling, thrift shopping, dancing, and floating on the river.

More information about Nancy and her work is available at her website:
https://www.nancyljohnston.com

Made in the USA
Las Vegas, NV
09 December 2024

13694169R00136